T0195304

CROSSING THE AMERICAN HEALTH CARE CHASM

CROSSING THE AMERICAN HEALTH CARE CHASM

Finding the Path to Bipartisan Collaboration in National Health Care Policy

DONALD A. BARR, MD, PhD

JOHNS HOPKINS UNIVERSITY PRESS | *Baltimore*

Johns Hopkins University Press
2715 North Charles Street
Baltimore, Maryland 21218-4363
www.press.jhu.edu

Library of Congress Cataloging-in-Publication Data

Names: Barr, Donald A., author.
Title: Crossing the American health care chasm : finding the path to bipartisan
    collaboration in national health care policy / Donald A. Barr.
Description: Baltimore : Johns Hopkins University Press, [2021] |
    Includes bibliographical references and index.
Identifiers: LCCN 2020041837 | ISBN 9781421441337 (hardcover ; alk. paper) |
    ISBN 9781421441344 (ebook)
Subjects: MESH: United States. Patient Protection and Affordable Care Act. |
    Health Policy | Health Care Reform | United States
Classification: LCC RA445 | NLM WA 540 AA1 | DDC 362.10973—dc23
LC record available at https://lccn.loc.gov/2020041837

A catalog record for this book is available from the British Library.

*Special discounts are available for bulk purchases of this book. For more information,
please contact Special Sales at specialsales@jh.edu.*

Johns Hopkins University Press uses environmentally friendly book materials,
including recycled text paper that is composed of at least 30 percent post-consumer
waste, whenever possible.

CONTENTS

In the weeks leading up to the November 2020 elections, the United States found itself in a deep partisan divide over the way we deliver health care to the American people. While the rapid spread of the COVID-19 pandemic in early 2020 added to its complexity, the divide existed well before the pandemic. The 10 years following enactment of the Patient Protection and Affordable Care Act (ACA) involved a series of partisan efforts either to revoke or to weaken the act. In December 2019, only a month before COVID-19 began its spread, a federal appeals court ruled that a central component of the act was unconstitutional. The Supreme Court heard an appeal of that ruling a week after the election and is expected to issue its ruling in spring or summer of 2021.

In an Op-Ed published in the *New York Times* in April 2020, Susan Rice, former US ambassador to the United Nations and national security advisor to President Obama, reported, "The coronavirus has laid bare our domestic divisions, unequal economy, and glaring racial and socioeconomic disparities as well as the fragility of our democracy." That same month, Jaime S. King, the associate dean and professor of law at the UC Hastings College of the Law, published an article in the *New England Journal of Medicine* titled, "Covid-19 and the Need for Health Care Reform." In the article Professor King argued that "the patchwork way we govern and pay for health care is unraveling in this time of crisis, leaving millions of people vulnerable and requiring swift, coordinated political action to ensure access to affordable care" (2020, p. 1).

Professors David R. Williams of Harvard and Lisa A. Cooper of Johns Hopkins (2020) referenced other types of pandemics that predated COVID-19: "COVID-19 is a magnifying glass that has highlighted the larger pandemic of racial/ethnic disparities in health. For more than 100 years research has documented that African American and Native American individuals have shorter life spans and more illness than white persons" (Williams and Cooper 2020, p. 2478). Monica Hooper and her colleagues from the National Institute of Minority Health and Health Disparities underscored the point that, rather than creating these racial disparities, COVID-19 simply exacerbated them. "The pandemic has shone a spotlight on health disparities and created an opportunity to address the causes underlying these inequities. The most pervasive disparities are observed among African American and Latino individuals, and where data exist, American Indian, Alaska Native, and Pacific Islander populations" (Hooper, Nápoles, and Pérez-Stable 2020, p. 2466).

These inequalities in outcomes, as well as the vulnerability cited by Professor King, are untoward consequences of the COVID-19 crisis, but they are not new. They are simply extensions of the vulnerabilities and disparities that existed before the advent of the SARS-CoV-2 virus.

Bartsch and colleagues (2020) estimated the cost of providing hospital care nationally to those with COVID-19 at between $163 billion and $654 billion, depending on what percentage of the population becomes infected and requires hospital care. This would be on top of the continuous increase in US health care costs we have witnessed in recent years. Even though the original ACA legislation was projected to lead to a reduction in health expenditures, Antos and Capretta (2020, p. 2) reported, "National health expenditure data show that such savings have not been realized." They underscore that, following the years of the Trump administration's efforts to disrupt the ACA, "health care costs continue to rise, and efforts to promote greater efficiency in health care delivery have been disappointing. A true revolution is needed if we are to address the real long-standing problems of cost, quality, and access to appropriate care" (p. 6).

What are the chances of our country realizing "a true revolution" in health care? In her *New York Times* Op-Ed, Ambassador Susan Rice suggested that such a revolution may indeed be possible: "As we struggle through the COVID-19 crisis . . . we must ask again how we can emerge a more just, equitable and cohesive nation." Rice suggests that there is indeed a way out of this conundrum, and that way involves an aspect of American society fundamental since its inception. "Yet in this moment of crisis, thankfully, nothing can happen without bipartisan compromise . . . [W]e can again emerge from profound crisis with renewed national strength and unity."

With this book, I hope to support Ambassador Rice's perspective. With the election of Joseph Biden as President, we once again have the opportunity to put aside rigid partisanship and "restore the soul of America," as Biden pledged in his speech following his election. We have been able to achieve bipartisanship at other critical points in American history. We can do it again now. I offer a way that we can bridge the wide chasm that has developed over where we should take our system of health care.

CROSSING THE AMERICAN HEALTH CARE CHASM

Introduction

IN JUNE 2019, two articles appeared side-by-side in the *New England Journal of Medicine*. The first was by Blendon, Benson, and McMurtry, who reported their analysis of more than a dozen national opinion polls addressing current health care issues. The biggest issue for the American public is health care costs, with more than two-thirds of respondents indicating that reducing those costs should be a top national priority. While those on different sides of the political spectrum agreed on this general issue, they did *not* agree on how to address it. Among Republicans, 61% believed private health insurance companies would be better at reducing costs, while 65% of Democrats considered this the job of government. Among those respondents preferring a government response, 63% of Republicans indicated that state government was best suited to take on health care costs, while 69% of Democrats thought this was the federal government's responsibility.

This partisan schism has been evident since early in the Obama administration. In 2017, a staunchly Republican Senate came within one vote of repealing much of the Affordable Care Act (ACA). The Trump administration consistently chipped away at the act through a series of administrative changes. With the leadership of the House in Democratic hands following the 2018 elections, there seemed little chance of any collaborative solution to the challenges confronting our health care system.

In the second article, titled "Sitting in Limbo—Obamacare under Divided Government," Jonathan Oberlander concluded that "intensifying partisan polarization in Congress has made it more difficult to forge compromise, leading to more legislative deadlock . . . The ideological chasm between Democrats and Republicans in Congress makes it difficult to find common ground on policy" (2019, p. 2486).

Has the schism between Republicans and Democrats over issues of health care become a chasm? What is the difference between a schism and a chasm? The *Oxford English Dictionary* (*OED*) defines a schism as "a division into mutually opposing parties of a body of persons that have previously acted in concert." By comparison, a chasm is "a wide and profound difference of character or position, a breach of relations, feelings, interests."

The *OED* offers a second meaning for the word chasm: "A large and deep rent, cleft, or fissure in the surface of the earth." When I think about the "wide and profound difference of character or position" that currently exists in our government and more widely in our populace, the image of a large and deep fissure is what comes to mind.

There was a time in the late twentieth century when Republicans and Democrats in Congress worked together to arrive at bipartisan solutions to major national health care problems. Although the gap in the late 1940s between President Harry S. Truman and conservative Republicans in Congress (and their supporters in the American Medical Association [AMA]) over the issue of national health insurance clearly qualified as a chasm, by the mid-1960s, President Lyndon B. Johnson and his colleague Congressman Wilbur Mills, a conservative Democrat from Arkansas, were able to work collaboratively to pass Medicare and Medicaid. In attaining this milestone in American health care, Democrats, Republicans, and even the American Medical Association came to an agreement on the issue of health care for vulnerable populations.

Bipartisanship was to reappear in 1997 with the passage of the State Children's Health Insurance Program (SCHIP). Only a few years earlier,

President Bill Clinton's efforts at national health care reform came to naught when Newt Gingrich and his fellow Republicans took control of the House of Representatives following the November 1994 elections. Much of the responsibility, however, lay with Bill and Hillary Clinton and their plan to employ a White House task force to design the reform legislation and deliver the final legislation to Congress for review and approval. As the Clintons learned, that's not the way Congress works. The failure of the Clinton health plan stemmed from this tactical error more than it reflected a true schism between the political parties.

Beginning early in his administration, President Barack Obama laid out the broad outlines of his plan for health care reform, but he left it to Congress to write the actual legislation to carry it out. With Democrats controlling both houses of Congress, he let congressional leaders know that they needed to pass the final legislation *before* the midterm elections of 2010, to avoid the same pitfall President Clinton had encountered. A group of moderate Republicans began to work collaboratively with their Democratic colleagues to draft legislation that had a good chance of gaining bipartisan support. An ad hoc committee of three Democratic senators and three Republican senators, all members of the Senate Finance Committee, began developing the outline of reform legislation. This "Gang of Six," as the group came to be known, held a series of about 30 meetings, with the goal of drafting legislation that would have the support of most Democrats and at least some Republicans.

After several months of bipartisan discussion and cooperation, Democratic leaders in Congress began pressing for a vote on a final legislation. The death of Senator Edward Kennedy, long a leading Democrat in the area of health care reform, led to a short-term appointment of another Democrat from Massachusetts to replace him in the Senate. That move allowed the Democrats to maintain a filibuster-proof, 60-vote majority, and the Senate passed the ACA at the end of December 2009.

In January 2010, a special election in Massachusetts to fill Ted Kennedy's seat resulted in a Republican win. Republicans, now with 41 votes in the Senate, were able to mount a filibuster to block the Democratic efforts to enact the ACA, at least in the Senate, following review by a House/Senate conference committee of any changes made by the House. The House of Representatives does not allow filibusters. Accordingly, the only option open to Democrats was for the House to approve without amendment the version of the ACA that the Senate had passed in December.

The Democratic leadership in the House agreed to do this, on the condition that the Senate would then approve some modifications to the ACA generated by the House under the reconciliation process "by which Congress changes existing laws to conform tax and spending levels to the levels set in a budget resolution," as defined by the rules of the US Senate (n.d.). As such, reconciliation legislation is not subject to a filibuster and needs only 51 votes in the Senate to become law.

On March 21, 2010, the House approved the original ACA legislation passed by the Senate. That same day, the House passed the Health Care and Education Reconciliation Act of 2010, the addendum to the ACA containing the changes the House had insisted on as a condition of passing the Senate version of ACA. On March 25, the Senate passed this reconciliation act with some minor amendments. That same day, the House approved this amended version. On March 23, President Obama signed the ACA legislation into law. On March 30, he signed the reconciliation act into law. President Obama and congressional Democrats had succeeded where previous administrations had repeatedly failed.

Perhaps not surprisingly, congressional Republicans were not at all happy with their exclusion from the process of drafting of the final legislation. Some Republicans were livid. The bipartisanship attendant to the drafting of the ACA during the early months of the Obama administration rapidly morphed into a schism between congressional Democrats and Republicans. The schism widened when Republicans took control of the House after the November 2010 midterm elections. House Republicans tried repeatedly, and unsuccessfully, to repeal major portions of the ACA. This schism has only become starker after Republicans took control of the Senate in the 2014 elections and President Donald J. Trump was elected in 2016. What we are now facing is a large and deep fissure in the surface of the earth inhabited by politics, a deep political chasm.

How will this chasm affect American health care? This is a question well worth considering. Health care costs continue to rise, impacting millions of insured Americans with out-of-pocket costs they often can barely afford. Reed Abelson (2019) reported in the *New York Times* that, while employer-provided health insurance covers more than 150 million people in the United States, the rising premiums and associated deductibles are making it harder and harder for many employees to afford that coverage. Abelson concluded that "the current system results in a schism between those who have good employer coverage and those who do not."

The data Abelson cites are consistent with the results of the poll by Blendon, Benson, and McMurtry (2019, p. 2491) cited above, in which the authors conclude, "This debate tracks with the partisan divide: Republicans generally believe that private health insurance and state governments would be more effective at reducing costs, whereas Democrats tend to support efforts by government, especially the federal government, to address the problem."

In the leadup to the 2020 elections, many Democratic candidates voiced their support for different forms of Medicare expansion as an alternative. Abelson cited a recent poll from the *Wall Street Journal* and NBC News showing that 56% of Americans are opposed to moving to a government-run system such as "Medicare for All." Despite these numbers, some candidates were advocating for Medicare for All. Others were championing for a narrower expansion of Medicare only to certain groups, such as those over age 50. However, as described by Larry Levitt of the Kaiser Family Foundation (2019), "Any differences among the Democratic candidates on health care are dwarfed by the wide gulf that separates all of them from President Trump." It seems readily apparent that this wide gulf has become a chasm that now separates Democrats and Republicans over the issue of health care.

How did this chasm open up? What was it about the schism that developed between Republicans and Democrats following the last-minute enactment of the ACA and the reconciliation bill that accompanied it? In their effort to "repeal and replace" the ACA, what actions have Republicans taken that gradually yet consistently widened the initial schism into the deep chasm we now confront? These are the issues this book will address.

Outline of the Book

In chapter 1, I describe the health care chasm that yawned when Harry Truman became president following the death of Franklin D. Roosevelt. Truman was deeply committed to enacting a plan for national health insurance, as Roosevelt had initially proposed in the 1930s. While Truman had the support of three Democratic senators who drafted legislation to do just that, on the other side of the chasm stood the American Medical Association, which accused President Truman of supporting a form of socialized medicine. By the late 1950s, this concern had lessened, and labor unions began advocating for government-sponsored health insurance for seniors.

The House Ways and Means Committee, under the leadership of Representative Mills, began exploring possible legislation to enact health care for seniors. In 1960, an interim plan, the Kerr-Mills Act, was approved by Congress and signed by President Dwight D. Eisenhower, providing federal subsidies to states to help pay for health care needed by seniors in poverty. The election of President John F. Kennedy in 1960 led to renewed discussion of adopting a broad program of health insurance for seniors. However, a coalition of conservative southern Democrats was able to block congressional approval. Only after the death of President Kennedy, the assumption of the presidency by Lyndon Johnson, and the expanded Democratic congressional majorities following the 1964 elections was the Democratic leadership able to bring health insurance to the forefront of discussion. The chapter concludes with a description of the "three-layer cake" compromise, attained under the leadership of President Johnson and Chairman Mills, which led to final approval of Medicare and Medicaid.

Chapter 2 traces the bipartisanship built over the four decades following the passage of Medicare and Medicaid. During President Jimmy Carter's administration, the national focus was on controlling hospital costs. Rather than imposing government controls, Congress enacted a series of laws that relied on private-sector organizations to monitor hospital cost and quality. Under the Reagan administration, Congress fundamentally changed the way hospitals are paid under Medicare to a system of fixed, prospective payment rates based on the condition of the patient receiving treatment. In the year before President Ronald Reagan was elected, a strongly bipartisan Congress also passed the Bayh-Dole Act, fundamentally changing the patent rights to discoveries made with federal funding.

President Clinton was unsuccessful in gaining approval for the Health Security Act he proposed. Even those who worked under White House direction to draft the act agreed after the fact that the failure to pass the bill was largely due to the manner in which they wrote the proposed legislation, rather than partisan opposition to the plan. A few years after the defeat of the Health Security Act, President Clinton was able to build strong bipartisan support in Congress for creation of the State Children's Health Insurance Program, extending federally financed health insurance to children in families with incomes up to twice the poverty line.

The congressional bipartisanship that passed SCHIP weakened under President George W. Bush when he proposed pharmaceutical coverage under Medicare, combined with substantially enhanced payments to private managed-care companies who enrolled Medicare beneficiaries. The law was approved by narrow margins in Congress, split largely along party lines. However, the parties in Congress came together again in 2007 to extend SCHIP and to expand it to families with incomes up to 300% of poverty. Despite strong bipartisan support in Congress, President Bush vetoed this law, criticizing it for providing health insurance to families who should instead be paying for the coverage themselves. Congress tried twice to override President Bush's veto, coming up only a few votes short.

Chapter 3 describes the efforts during the first 12 months of the Obama administration to pass two crucial pieces of legislation: the renewal of SCHIP that President Bush had previously vetoed and the development and final passage of the Affordable Care Act. There was broad bipartisan support for the former. It took Congress only about a month not only to renew funding for children's health care but also to expand eligibility to families with incomes up to 300% of the federal poverty line (FPL). Now referred to simply as CHIP, President Obama signed the legislation about two weeks after taking office.

Once CHIP was approved, President Obama then focused on his campaign pledge to accomplish comprehensive health care reform. Taking a clear message from the failure of the Clinton administration's health care proposal, President Obama left it largely up to Congress to draft the legislation. The House and Senate Democratic leadership introduced their version of the reform legislation in July for review by the appropriate committees. The House approved its final version in early November. The review and approval process in the House was largely partisan, having lost much of the sense of bipartisanship early on.

The Senate adopted more of a bipartisan process in crafting its version of the legislation, with senators from both parties on the Finance Committee holding a series of collaborative meetings. The untimely death of Senator Ted Kennedy resulted in the Democrats facing the potential of losing their 60-vote filibuster-proof majority in mid-January. Accordingly, the Senate approved its version of the reform legislation on December 24. A complex process unfolded, with two pieces of legislation finally passing, one of which was structured as a reconciliation bill. The process that congressional Democrats had to follow in order to avoid a looming Republican filibuster in the Senate angered many congressional Republicans. When President Obama signed the final bills into law in March 2010, any sense of congressional bipartisanship regarding health reform legislation had largely been lost.

In chapter 4, I examine the repeated efforts of congressional Republicans and their allies in states with Republican leadership either to repeal or to substantially weaken the ACA. On the same day President Obama signed the ACA into law, the State of Florida filed a lawsuit challenging the constitutionality of the individual mandate written into the law. Several other states joined in the lawsuit, as well as the National Federation of Independent Business. The plaintiffs also challenged the constitutionality of the expansion of Medicaid eligibility mandated by the ACA. The lawsuit was heard by the US Supreme Court, which upheld the mandate but made Medicaid expansion optional for the states.

Under Republican leadership following the 2010 elections, the House repeatedly passed measures to repeal the ACA. The Senate, still under Democratic control, blocked each of these bills. Largely out of frustration, a group of private citizens with funding from an activist conservative organization filed another lawsuit to invalidate the extension of premium tax credits to individuals and families who obtain their health insurance coverage through Healthcare.gov, the federal exchange. Once again, the Supreme Court overturned lower court decisions that would have blocked payment of these credits. In response to these legal setbacks, the Republican House of Representatives filed its own lawsuit against the Obama administration to block certain other payments under the ACA.

In the elections in November 2014, Republicans increased their majority in the House and took over leadership in the Senate. With control of both houses of Congress, Republicans were able to pass a law repealing most aspects of the ACA. As expected, President Obama vetoed it, and Republicans failed in their attempt to override. The intensity of the dispute over the ACA only intensified as the country approached November 2016.

The election of President Trump in 2016 begins chapter 5, which then discusses the executive order he issued on the day of his inauguration instructing his administration to seek prompt repeal of the ACA. With continued Republican majorities in the House and the Senate, the efforts to repeal the ACA began in earnest.

By early May, the House had passed its version of repeal—the American Health Care Act. Rather than vote on the House version of repeal legislation, the Senate developed its own version—the Better Care Reconciliation Act. The Congressional Budget Office predicted the probable impacts of both. Each bill would have substantially increased the number of people without health insurance, considerably raised health insurance premiums in the private market, and reduced the federal deficit by different amounts.

When it came up for a vote in the Senate, the Better Care Reconciliation Act failed by a vote of 43-57. Nine Republicans joined all Senate Democrats in defeating it. Senate majority leader Mitch McConnell then introduced alternative legislation to weaken rather than repeal the

ACA—the Health Care Freedom Act. When it came up for a vote, three Republican senators joined all 48 Democrats in rejecting the legislation, with Senator John McCain casting his now iconic "thumbs-down" vote.

The multiple failures to repeal the ACA by a secretive process that excluded any participation by congressional Democrats drew criticism from a number of commentators. These included the three Republican senators who voted against the Health Care Freedom Act. These senators urged President Trump and congressional Republicans to initiate a bipartisan discussion with Democrats to modify the ACA in a way that could gain broad support.

Rather than following this recommendation, President Trump and congressional Republicans began attacking the ACA in ways that only widened the schism between the parties. Chapter 6 considers how congressional Republicans focused their efforts to disrupt ACA financing of two programs: the payment of cost-sharing reductions (CSRs) and the payment for risk corridors.

Under the ACA, in addition to qualifying for federal tax credits to help pay premiums for insurance purchased through the exchanges, individuals and families with incomes between 100% and 250% of FPL had a cap placed on the amount they would have to spend out of pocket for deductibles, copayments, and prescription drugs. The ACA promised that the federal government would reimburse insurance companies for these CSRs. However, the ACA did not include a specific authorization to fund these reimbursements. The Republican House of Representatives sued the Obama administration to block these payments. Once President Trump came into office, he agreed to stop them. The result was a destabilization of the health insurance markets nationally. Ironically, as described in the chapter, the result was a substantial increase in federal expenditures, rather than the expected decrease.

The ACA also promised to cover the costs of any excess losses insurance companies encountered during the first three years of the ACA marketplaces—referred to as the risk corridor. The Republican House of Representatives also blocked funding for these payments. As a consequence, insurance companies experienced an aggregate loss of

$12 billion during this time, and numerous insurance companies left the market. Many of the new nonprofit co-op health insurance plans that were established as part of the ACA were bankrupted. The insurance companies filed a class-action suit to recover their losses. After trials in lower courts, the Supreme Court heard oral arguments in the suit December 2019. The court issued its ruling in April 2020, finding that the federal government is fully responsible for $12.2 billion in outstanding risk corridor payments.

Chapter 7 addresses a number of efforts congressional Republicans and President Trump have taken to further weaken the ACA. An important step by Congress was to revoke the tax penalty assessed under the individual mandate created by the ACA. With no penalty for going without health insurance, the Congressional Budget Office predicted that several million younger and relatively healthy individuals would drop their health insurance coverage, leading to significantly increased premiums for those who maintain coverage through the ACA exchanges. The repeal of the individual mandate tax penalty also resulted in a legal challenge to the constitutionality of the entire ACA, as addressed in the following chapter.

President Trump has used administrative changes under executive order in an attempt to further weaken the ACA. In October 2017, after the failure of Republican efforts in Congress to repeal the ACA, President Trump issued an executive order to alter the rules that govern health insurance sold on the ACA exchanges. The rule authorized a new form of health insurance organized by groups of small employers referred to as an association health plan. It would also authorize the issuance of health insurance policies that were for periods less than one year. While both types of plans would be substantially cheaper than plans sold in the individual market through the ACA, they would also be substantially less comprehensive in their coverage. Both were predicted to attract principally younger, healthier individuals, resulting in further increases in ACA marketplace premiums.

Legal actions taken by several states have for now blocked the issuance of these new types of noncompliant plans. In addition, several states have imposed regulations to either restrict or prohibit their issuance.

Two additional steps to weaken or invalidate the ACA are the subject of chapter 8. Even though the expansion of Medicaid under the ACA was ruled to be optional for the states, a growing number of states that have elected to expand Medicaid requested and were granted permission by the Trump administration to impose work requirements of a minimum of 20 hours per week on non-elderly, nondisabled adults covered by Medicaid. Certain adults who are caring for very young children are exempted. In addition, other types of activities, such as engaging in community service or enrolling in school, would be an option for those unable to find work.

Kentucky was the first to be granted permission under a Section 1115 waiver to impose work requirements on its Medicaid recipients. Soon after it was granted by the Department of Health and Human Services, a federal district court ruled the work requirements invalid. This ruling was subsequently applied to several other states. One state, Arkansas, had already implemented its work requirement, leading to more than 18,000 Medicaid recipients losing their coverage. The court ruling against Kentucky and the other states was expanded to include Arkansas, so those recipients regained their coverage. The Trump administration appealed this ruling. The appeals court upheld the lower court's ruling in February 2020, finding that the Medicaid work requirements were "arbitrary and capricious."

Perhaps the most serious threat to the ACA is from a decision issued by a federal district court judge in *Texas v. United States*. Following the revocation of the individual mandate tax penalty by the Republican Congress, the text of the individual mandate requirement to maintain health insurance itself remained part of the ACA. The Supreme Court had previously ruled that this part of the mandate was not permissible under the Constitution. The lawsuit filed in Texas asked the judge to rule that, since one portion of the ACA legislation violated the Constitution, the entire law must therefore be unconstitutional. The Texas court agreed with this reasoning but stayed enforcement of the decision pending appeal. The case then moved to the appeals court, which ruled in December 2019 that the insurance mandate without the tax penalty was unconstitutional and referred the case back to the circuit court to determine which other parts of the ACA would be affected by this ruling. In March 2020, the Supreme Court agreed to hear the case. The hearing was held on November 10, one week after the 2020 elections.

Largely as a result of these various efforts undertaken over a period of nearly a decade either to weaken or to repeal the ACA, a deep sense of rancor has emerged between most Democrats and Republicans in Congress. Indeed, the timing of the impeachment process charging President Trump with abuse of power and obstruction of Congress only intensified this rancor. How will it be possible for those on either side of this political and cultural chasm to reestablish trust and communication and to take mutually agreed-upon steps to assure that the ACA, either in its current form or in a modified version, can assure nearly all Americans of access to high-quality, affordable health insurance?

Chapter 9 takes on this challenge. In it I suggest a way to bridge the chasm that has grown between the different factions in the debate over US health care. I use the metaphor of a bridge made of ropes fashioned from hay, such as the Q'eswachaka Rope Bridge. This bridge is built through the close collaboration of indigenous groups on both sides of the Apurimac Canyon in Peru. I then describe a series of policy "ropes" politicians on both sides of the health care chasm could fashion together to address problems that have been shown to have broad bipartisan public support.

In the final chapter, I provide a summary of the issues raised in the book. I offer my analysis of what has worked over the years in maintaining a sense of bipartisan collaboration in American health policy. What lessons have we learned? What more recent factors have led to the cultural and ideological divide over health care reform that we now confront? Is this divide fundamentally different from those of earlier points in history? I suggest that we can learn from previous bipartisan efforts to reestablish a sense of trust and collaboration in order to address our current health care problems.

I hope, as you are delving into the specific issues and questions each chapter describes, you will ask yourself whether you believe it is feasible for our society to reestablish a sense of collaborative commitment to the common good. Perhaps, in hoping for a return of national bipartisanship, I am being quixotic. Which aspect of "quixotic," though, might you apply to my efforts? The *OED* offers two definitions:

1. naively idealistic, unrealistic, impracticable; or
2. visionary.

I will leave it to you, the reader, to apply to my work the quality you see as more appropriate.

ONE

Bipartisanship in Health Care during the Late Twentieth Century

THE CURRENT dilemma confronting the US health care system is not the first we have experienced as a chasm in social and political thinking regarding health care. Those who have studied the history of health care in the mid-twentieth century are well aware of the political chasm Harry Truman faced in his attempts to create a national system of health care.

Franklin Roosevelt initially considered including health care for seniors as an added benefit of the Social Security system he established in the 1930s. The American Medical Association had sufficient influence to nix that proposal, threatening to block passage of Social Security entirely. Fully appreciating the political power wielded at that time by the AMA, Roosevelt deferred, dropping the health care component of the new retirement benefit system.

Part of the new Social Security system was a national Social Security Board established by the legislation to oversee administration of the new system. During the waning years of World War II, members of the board began exploring options for adding a health care benefit for seniors who qualified to receive a retirement cash benefit. Responding to the Social Security Board's lead, in 1945 Democratic senators Robert F. Wagner from New York and James Murray from Montana and Democratic representative John D. Dingell from Michigan introduced a bill in Congress that would make government-sponsored health insurance available to all Americans, not just those receiving a Social Security pension.

As described in the history published by the Social Security Administration (n.d.):

> As its drafters and sponsors had expected, the Wagner-Murray-Dingell bill signaled the beginning of the political debate that would come to a climax in the postwar years. In the ensuing months, the battle lines began to form. Organized labor, the National Farmers Union, and several other organizations declared their support; the AMA-linked "National Physicians' Committee for the Extension of Medical Service" began organizing against it . . . The physicians were joined by a revitalized Insurance Economics Society of America, the Pharmaceutical Manufacturers' Association, and other groups.

The first iteration of the Wagner-Murray-Dingell bill never made it out of committee, either in the Senate or the House. Not to be deterred, President Franklin Roosevelt planned to add his influence to the effort. In his budget message delivered to Congress in January 1945, Roosevelt called for an expansion of Social Security to include medical care. Unfortunately, Roosevelt's death in April 1945 set this goal back, leaving it to President Truman to take over the effort.

Following the defeat of the Japanese and the end of World War II, President Truman sent a message to Congress calling for comprehensive insurance benefits covering medical, dental, hospital, and nursing services, reforms included in the Wagner-Murray-Dingell bill (Marmor 1973). The plan, commonly referred to as National Health Insurance, would be available to all workers and their families, and would be financed by a 3% payroll tax shared equally by the employer and the employee. Federal grants to states would subsidize the insurance for those who were retired or unemployed. Doctors would be free to elect to participate in the plan or not. Once again, the proposed bill never made it beyond congressional committees.

The Congress elected in 1946 following the end of the war had a substantially conservative perspective, especially in the House Ways and

Means Committee. As described in the Social Security Administration history, "Taken alone, these factors would not have posed an insurmountable obstacle to a health-insurance measure had there not also been a deep cleavage on the issue between major interest groups in the community" (n.d.). Conservatives in Congress refused even to hold hearings on the Wagner-Murray-Dingell bill in the House Ways and Means Committee.

In 1948, President Truman achieved reelection, and Democrats won majorities in both houses of Congress. Once again, the Wagner-Murray-Dingell bill was reintroduced, but conservative intransigence remained among many southern Democrats, as the bill would have expanded health insurance to Blacks in the South. Once again, the bill never made it out of committee for an actual floor vote.

By then, the AMA had developed a deep concern over Truman's efforts. In December 1948, it convened an urgent meeting of its House of Delegates, which voted to assess each member nationally a fee of $25 to finance a national campaign against the bill, which the AMA saw as threatening to enslave physicians under a national health care program. In the era of growing anti-communist concern, the AMA repeatedly described Truman's efforts at reform as advocating "socialized medicine."

Robert Ball, the Social Security commissioner at the time of the enactment of Medicare, characterized the AMA's opposition to the Wagner-Murray-Dingell bill in these terms (1995, p. 64): "The AMA's opposition approached hysteria. Members were assessed dues for the first time to create a $3.5 million war chest—very big money for the times—with which the association conducted an unparalleled campaign of vituperation against the advocates of national health insurance. The AMA also exerted strict discipline over the few of its members who took an 'unethical' position favoring the government program." As described by Marmor (1973, p. 13), "The AMA took the issue of 'socialized medicine' to both the primary and general elections, and their propaganda was credited with the defeat of the Senate's firmest supporters of health insurance."

With the outbreak of the Korean War, the nation became preoccupied with anti-communism, Senator Joseph McCarthy, Republican of Wisconsin, leading the effort. It was easy for the AMA to portray their efforts to defeat attempts at national health insurance as part of anti-Communism. President Truman essentially gave up on his efforts to put in place national health insurance.

With the repeated defeat of the Wagner-Murray-Dingell bill's proposal for national health insurance for all Americans, the focus of discussions among those in government began to turn toward expanding health insurance options for seniors. Oscar Ewing, administrator of the Federal Security Agency, the agency established in 1939 to oversee Social Security, began to address the growing number of seniors in the United States. Based on a proposal by I. S. Falk of the federal Bureau of Research and Statistics, Ewing offered his support for providing health insurance to Social Security beneficiaries.

In 1950, the census counted 12 million people age 65 or over. Among these seniors, two-thirds had annual incomes of less than $1,000, and only 1 in 8 had any form of health insurance. In 1952, the annual report of the Social Security Administration included a recommendation that Congress establish federally funded health insurance for Social Security beneficiaries.

Among the principal beneficiaries of the expanding private health insurance market that followed World War II were members of labor unions. These unions began to campaign for making health insurance a retirement benefit under Social Security. In 1957, the executive council of the AFL-CIO adopted a policy that committed the 14-million-member labor federation to promoting the establishment of government health insurance for seniors. The American Nurses Association also endorsed this policy.

In 1957, Representative Aime J. Forand, a Democrat from Rhode Island, introduced in the House a proposal for health insurance for Social Security beneficiaries. The Forand bill began to gather growing support, principally among congressional Democrats. While no action was taken on it for three years, by 1960 Congressman Forand had secured enough votes for the bill to be considered by the House Ways and Means Committee. Although the bill was defeated by a substantial margin, the action represented the first formal vote on the issue of health insurance for seniors ever taken by Ways and Means.

The success in getting the committee at least to consider the Forand bill was followed by growing enthusiasm among the Democratic leadership in both the House and the Senate. House Speaker Sam Rayburn of Texas and Senate majority leader Lyndon B. Johnson, also of Texas, both backed the proposal. Representative Wilbur Mills, a Democrat from Arkansas, had become chairman of the House Ways and Means Committee. In light of the growing support for the Forand bill yet acknowledging that it was insufficient to attain full congressional approval for the proposed program, Mills began to work on finding a compromise.

In 1959, Arthur Flemming, secretary of Health, Education and Welfare under the Eisenhower administration, proposed an alternative arrangement under which the federal government would provide grants funded out of general revenues to subsidize individual states in acquiring private health insurance for low-income seniors. Vice President Richard M. Nixon gave this alternative approach his personal blessing and garnered the president's endorsement of the plan.

In June 1960, Chairman Mills came up with a compromise. With the backing of the AMA, Mills proposed expanding the existing program of medical payments provided under the state-run welfare programs. His plan would create a new category called "medical indigency" for low-income elderly people who needed help paying their medical bills but who otherwise would not qualify for welfare in their state.

Mills's proposal received bipartisan congressional buy-in. Referred to as H.R. 12580, it was rapidly reviewed and approved by the Ways and Means Committee. With agreement for a rapid vote from the House Rules Committee, the bill was approved by the House of Representatives by a vote of 381-23.

The bill was then taken up by the Senate Finance Committee. Democratic senator Robert Kerr of Oklahoma became one of the principal sponsors of the bill in the Senate, and the Finance Committee elected to rename it the Kerr-Mills bill. The committee approved the bill by a vote of 12-5 and sent it to the full Senate for consideration. During the Senate debate, a Republican proposal for a more generous subsidy to the states for private health insurance and a Democratic plan for direct federal provision of health insurance to Social Security beneficiaries were both defeated. As a compromise between these divergent proposals, the Kerr-Mills bill passed by a margin of 91-2.

The principal objective of the Kerr-Mills Act was to provide funding for "anyone over 65 whose resources were insufficient to meet his medical expenses" (Marmor 1973, p. 35). The act provided for a comprehensive range of benefits for those who were eligible based on medical need, including physician's services, hospital care, nursing home care, prescription drugs, and dental care. The money for these services came from a combination of federal and matching state funds. The federal government would pay between 50% and 80% of the costs, with the state paying the balance. The higher federal percentage would go to lower-income states. The plan was administered by the states, with each setting its own eligibility standard.

Relatively few states established programs for providing benefits under Kerr-Mills. At the end of the first year, "60% of the enrollees and almost 90% of the expenditures for the aged medically indigent were in three States: New York, Massachusetts, and California" (Moore and Smith 2005, p. 46). By 1963, 32 states were participating in the program. Nonetheless, 90% of the benefits were still going to 5 of the largest states—California, New York, Massachusetts, Michigan, and Pennsylvania. The aged population of these five states represented only 32% of the total population over 65 nationally (Marmor 1973).

Many of the other states that had adopted the program had placed strict limitations on the level of care provided. Nonetheless, Kerr-Mills had provided an alternative to the more generous benefits that had been proposed by many Democrats in Congress to provide health care for all Social Security beneficiaries regardless of income. Kerr-Mills also had the backing of the AMA.

The Road from Kerr-Mills to Medicare and Medicaid

The Kerr-Mills Act was approved by Congress in August 1960. At the same time, the presidential campaigns of John Kennedy and Richard Nixon were in full swing. Senator Kennedy, the Democratic candidate, continued to stump for government-financed health insurance for seniors as a central tenet of his campaign. Emerging victorious from the November elections, President Kennedy expressed his strong endorsement of the program he referred to as Medicare. Prior to his inauguration he established the Task Force on Health and Social Security for the American People. He appointed Professor Wilbur Cohen from the University of Michigan as chair. Acting rapidly, the task force published a report that recommended establishing a national hospital insurance program for seniors as part of Social Security.

Along with a Democratic president, the elections gave Democrats a majority in both the House of Representatives (260 seats to 175) and the Senate (64 seats to 36). Lyndon Johnson, the former Senate majority leader, was now Kennedy's vice president. Shortly after his inauguration, President Kennedy sent a special message to Congress on health care, voicing his commitment to the new Medicare plan. His administration also submitted a legislative proposal to Congress to enact Medicare. The bill was sponsored in the Senate by Clinton Anderson of New Mexico and in the House by Cecil King of California.

Despite a clear Democratic majority, in the 1960s a substantial proportion of Democrats in both the Senate and the House were from southern states. These southern Democrats tended to be more conservative than Democrats from other parts of the country. President Kennedy came to appreciate that a combination of southern Democrats and conservative Republicans carried sufficient weight in Congress to block passage of the proposed Medicare plan. Accordingly, he asked that Congress not hold a vote on the King-Anderson bill to avoid an early defeat. The plan was instead to focus on the 1962 elections with the hope of soliciting enough votes for passage in the next session of Congress.

While support for the King-Anderson bill was strong among many in Congress, as well as in public opinion nationally, there was one organization that was adamantly opposed to Medicare: the American Medical Association. "The AMA launched an 'all-out effort' against 'the most deadly challenge ever faced by the medical profession.' The AMA's campaign included distribution of several million pamphlets, numerous radio and TV commercials, a heavy speechmaking schedule by a 70-man speakers bureau, Operation Coffee Cup (an effort to generate constituent letters to Congressmen), and other grass-roots activity in opposition to Medicare" (Social Security Administration n.d.). The AMA was joined by the national Blue Cross Association in opposition.

Max Skidmore (1989) has described one of the most wide-reaching efforts by the AMA to block health care reform for seniors: "The Association fought on many fronts, but the most brilliant of all its opposition efforts was built on a phonograph record, 'Ronald Reagan Speaks out Against Socialized Medicine.'" At the time, Reagan was a well-recognized television personality who had not yet entered politics. Skidmore quotes a section of Reagan's commentary on the phonograph record. "One of the traditional methods of imposing statism or socialism on people has been by way of medicine. It's very easy to disguise a medical program as a humanitarian project" (p. 93). Reagan goes on to describe the Forand bill, under review by the House Ways and Means Committee, as one of the principal examples of just such a program.

On the other side of the widening debate, a new National Council of Senior Citizens was formed to promote the bill. Membership in the council included retirees from the United Auto Workers, United Steel Workers, International Ladies Garment Workers, and other labor organizations. Within a few months, the council had members representing more than 1 million retirees. The National Council of Senior Citizens was joined by the National Council of Churches in advancing Medicare. In January 1962, the American Hospital Association (AHA), which had previously opposed government involvement in the private market for health care, reversed its position. For the AHA, federal financial support for the hospital care provided to seniors was considered essential to the fiscal stability of hospitals.

At the same time the AHA was splitting from the AMA, several moderate Republicans also began to split from the more conservative members of the party. Despite efforts by the House Ways and Means Committee to bottle up the King-Anderson bill, the Kennedy administration turned to this group of Republican proponents, among whom Jacob Javits of New York took on a leadership role. While they did not gain formal endorsement for the legislation, the administration was able to identify a number of issues on which it and the senators were close enough for compromise. With the Kerr-Mills Act providing benefits to only a minority of seniors, mostly in a small group of states, there was a growing realization that the bill was insufficient to meet the need of seniors who needed hospital treatment. The group of senators led by Javits would have preferred a program under which seniors were able to enroll in Blue Cross or other private insurance, with financial assistance from the federal government for those who could not afford private coverage.

The Social Security Administration's History of the Evolution of Medicare (n.d.) refers to an important shift in the position taken by the AMA in response to Senate support for such a private insurance option: "In a magazine interview, AMA Executive Vice President F. J. L. Blasingame indicated that his organization might ultimately accept Federal subsidies for Blue Cross and Blue Shield coverage of the needy aged." So long as the program of health insurance for seniors was operated in the private sector and available based on financial need, the AMA might be able to acquiesce to it. The divide between the AMA and Democrats in Congress got a little narrower.

The period from 1960 to 1964 saw rapid increases in hospital costs in the private sector, and private insurers had no choice but also to increase premiums. Only about half of seniors had any form of health insurance, and only half of their plans were comprehensive enough to cover the full cost of hospitalization. This growing pressure on private insurance carriers was associated with growing support among some of the insurers, particularly smaller ones, for a government option such as Medicare. The waning opposition from the insurance industry and the openness to compromise on the part of the AMA encouraged the Kennedy administration and members of Congress to push harder to pass Medicare.

The 1962 elections saw the Democrats maintaining their majority in the House and expand their majority in the Senate. In the House, the Democratic leadership placed two new members on the Ways and Means Committee, both of whom had expressed support for Medicare. As the new Congress convened in 1963, representatives from the Kennedy administration began discussions with Representative Mills, chair of the committee, on possible compromises that might advance Medicare.

The Assassination of President Kennedy in November 1963 and the Rise of President Johnson

While he was alive, President Kennedy had strongly advocated for Medicare. As described above, his efforts were beginning to show some positive impacts, with congressional Republicans, the AMA, and the private insurance industry each showing movement toward collaborative discussions and compromise on how best to provide health insurance to seniors. Once Johnson was in place as president, he began pushing even harder to enact Medicare as well as other policy initiatives President Kennedy had pushed for.

By the summer of 1964, President Johnson had succeeded in getting the Senate Finance Committee to hold hearings on the King-Anderson bill, the original Medicare proposal submitted to Congress by President Kennedy in 1961. The bill failed the final vote in the committee by a 6-11 margin. The Democratic leadership was, however, successful in getting King-Anderson considered by the full Senate in the form of an amendment to another piece of legislation previously approved by the House. The amended bill, which included King-Anderson, was passed by the Senate in September by a vote of 49-44.

As the bill approved by the Senate had added this substantial change to the bill previously approved by the House, the legislation was sent to a House-Senate conference committee to find a compromise that could be accepted by both houses of Congress.

As chairman of Ways and Means, Mills was leader of the House component of the conference committee. Mills was opposed to the Medicare legislation and persuaded the House members of the committee to vote against including Medicare in the legislation by a 3-2 vote. The Senate members of the conference committee were equally adamant that the bill include Medicare, voting 4-3 to block committee approval of the bill without Medicare. By the first week in October, Mills announced to the public that the committee was deadlocked, and no compromise bill would be reported out to either house of Congress.

In announcing the failure of the conference committee to approve a bill that included Medicare, Chairman Mills indicated that he might be open to considering the proposal for Medicare during the next session of Congress in his committee. Thus, leading up to the 1964 elections, yet another powerful player indicated a move toward the middle and a willingness to compromise. In addition, national polls conducted prior to the election found that as many as two-thirds of voters were in favor of Medicare for seniors.

The 1964 Elections and Their Impact on Congress

Running against the far-right candidate Barry Goldwater, Lyndon Johnson was overwhelmingly reelected. Along with his victory came substantial gains for the Democrats in both houses of Congress: an additional 38 seats in the House, increasing their majority over Republicans to 295-140; and 2 in the Senate, bringing their majority to 68-32.

Recognizing the impact of these shifts, shortly after the election, Chairman Mills made a speech in which he announced, "I can support a pay-roll tax for financing health benefits just as I have supported a payroll tax for cash benefits" (Social Security Administration n.d.). Mills appeared to publicly acknowledge that, as a consequence of the election, the time had come for Medicare in some form.

As soon as the new session of Congress convened in 1965, Democrats were quick to reintroduce the King-Anderson bill into each house of Congress, and thus they were labeled H.R. 1 and S. 1. The Senate bill had 46 cosponsors, including three Republicans (Rosenblatt 2015, January 9).

With the reintroduction of the bill, President Johnson reached out to Wilbur Mills in an attempt to find common ground on Medicare. Johnson had indicated to Mills that passage of Medicare would give each of them an important place in the history of health care. As chairman of the Ways and Means Committee, Mills took personal responsibility for redrafting the bill into a form that could receive congressional approval. He focused his efforts on involving all the various parties that would be affected by Medicare in these discussions. By the end of January, Mills had initiated closed-door discussion of the bill by the committee.

While the AMA had earlier indicated potential assent to providing financial assistance for the needy aged to purchase private health insurance, it remained adamantly opposed to a government-run and government-financed health care benefit under Social Security, such as the one outlined in King-Anderson. In January 1965, the AMA leadership convened and laid out a national plan to oppose Medicare. However, "when spokesmen for the AMA invoked their fears of socialized medicine, they irritated committee members intent on working out practical matters, and Chairman Mills refused to consult AMA representatives in further sessions of the committee's officially unreported deliberations" (Marmor 1973, p. 62).

As described by Wilbur Cohen, the undersecretary of the Department of Health, Education and Welfare under President Johnson, "With the Johnson election victory, the AMA finally and belatedly decided to sponsor a counterproposal to Medicare" (1985, p. 6), which they named Eldercare. Under Eldercare, federal and state revenues would subsidize private insurance coverage for seniors, with the level of subsidy based on the senior's income. Two members of the House Ways and Means Committee, Sydney Herlong, a Democrat from Florida, and Thomas Curtis, a Republican from Missouri, submitted Eldercare legislation for consideration by the committee.

In February 1965, *JAMA: The Journal of the American Medical Association* reported, "The American Medical Association's House of Delegates voted to 'enthusiastically support' the Association's Eldercare program as embodied in the Herlong-Curtis bill and similar legislation now pending before Congress, and called on the Board of Trustees and two AMA Councils to investigate the possibility of expanding the Kerr-Mills program to provide aid for the medically needy of all ages" (AMA 1965, p. 32). The article also quotes Dr. Donovan Ward, president of the AMA, "as describing the Administration-backed King-Anderson bill—the so-called 'medicare' proposal—as 'a lure, not a cure, for the problems of the aged.'" The article also underscored the doctors' concern that the proposed Medicare program would provide only for hospital care and nursing home care but would not cover care provided by physicians.

In an article in the same issue of *JAMA*, titled "Are 200,000 Doctors Wrong?," Dr. Ward wrote (1965, p. 125):

> We have learned that a false promise, if it is given a fancy name, can be kept alive year after year—in spite of the truth—if drummed and promoted constantly among the people. Year after year, we have seen a piece of political quackery called medicare die in Congress, its promoters defeated by the sound judgment of the majority of the House Ways and Means Committee and by lack of support in our national legislature. After each of those beatings, we thought medicare would not dare show its false face again. We were wrong. It came back during the next election.

While opposing Medicare in the form it took in the King-Anderson bill, the AMA indicated its support for the approach taken by the Kerr-Mills bill from 1960. "The Herlong-Curtis eldercare bill can cover not only the cost of hospital care and nursing homes for the aged, but also payment of physicians and surgical and drug costs—which medicare would not do. It will be found that the Herlong-Curtis eldercare program will be financed by federal-state matching funds, expanding and strengthening the established Kerr-Mills Law" (p. 127). The AMA firmly backed a taxpayer-financed program for needy seniors to receive a comprehensive range of services, *including* payment for physicians' care.

An article published by Harold Brunn, executive secretary of the Minnesota State Medical Association, argued strongly in favor of Eldercare and against Medicare. "The introduction of the Herlong-Curtis Eldercare Bill (H.R. 3727) represents a breakthrough of historic importance to all citizens in the drive to provide people over 65 with a wide range of health care to meet their needs . . . Careful analysis of H.R. 3727 indicates that it will assure more benefits at less cost to the taxpayer, than any other measure for people 65 and over who need care and can't afford to pay for it" (Brunn 1965, p. 401).

While the Ways and Means Committee was discussing King-Anderson and Herlong-Curtis, yet another proposal was introduced by a group of House Republicans who did not favor the AMA's Eldercare proposal. Led by the new House minority leader, Gerald Ford, this group submitted a proposal for a system they referred to as "Bettercare." "They want the federal government to create a voluntary national insurance program, where people could buy private policies anywhere in the country. The federal government would provide funds out of annual appropriations for those too poor to afford insurance" (Rosenblatt 2015).

In his history *The Politics of Medicare*, Marmor (1973, p. 77) suggested, "The certainty that some Medicare bill would be enacted changed the incentives and disincentives facing former Medicare opponents. Suggesting a physicians' insurance alternative offered an opportunity for Republicans to cut their losses in the face of certain Democratic victory and to counteract public identification of Republican opposition with intransigent AMA opposition to Medicare."

It is worth noting that, although the Medicare bill would cover only hospital and nursing home care but not care provided by physicians, both Eldercare and Bettercare would include coverage for physician services. The explanation given by Commissioner Ball was that by excluding physician services, it would place no new government restrictions on the care provided by physicians. Since the FDR presidency, the AMA had expressed serious concerns regarding a government takeover of care.

By the end of February 1965, another organization had entered the national discussions over medical care. The AFL-CIO Executive Council publicly denounced the AMA's Eldercare plan as "unworkable" and filled with "empty promises" (Rosenblatt 2015, February 27). The labor unions argued for broad coverage for seniors that would include the hospital care covered under the Medicare proposal as well as care by doctors and pharmaceuticals.

Chairman Mills Surprises Everyone by Combining Three Rival Plans

At a meeting of the House Ways and Means Committee held in the first week of March, Mills announced his plan to combine the Johnson administration's Medicare proposal, the Bettercare proposal submitted by Gerald Ford and his Republican colleagues, and the Eldercare proposal by the AMA. "This new approach combines the President's plan to expand the Social Security payroll tax to directly pay hospitals for care provided to the elderly with a Republican plan to expand the voluntary private insurance system for this population. It also adds an AMA proposal to provide additional federal revenues to expand the Kerr-Mills program that helps the states pay for the medical bills of poor people" (Rosenblatt 2015, March 6).

The private correspondence between Mills and President Johnson that had been taking place since early January likely contributed to this bipartisan compromise drafted by Mills. Commissioner Ball recounted the process of negotiating a compromise legislation: "Part B was explicitly based on a private insurance plan, an Aetna plan for federal workers under the Federal Employees Health Benefits Program (FEHBP). It was to be voluntary, not paid-up insurance but financed by a current premium with half paid by the elderly who elected coverage and half by the federal government . . . We had only one weekend in which to try to adapt the Aetna plan to a government-run plan" (1995, p. 69).

Characterized in the press as a "three-layer cake," the compromise included key aspects of each of the three plans. "Mills had been opposed to the Medicare approach for years, but extensive private talks with Johnson and the results of the election persuaded this key congressional player that passage of a bill would become inevitable" (Rosenblatt 2015, March 27).

The Ways and Means Committee approved Chairman Mills's "three-layer cake" legislation by a vote of 17-8, along party lines. On March 25, Tom Wicker commented in an article in the *New York Times* on this major accomplishment (1965):

> The House Ways and Means Committee's approval of a plan for medical care for the aged tied to the Social Security system probably meant victory in a frustrating eight-year fight that began in 1957 . . . What happened in those eight years to turn repeated defeat into probable victory? The various answers illustrate an old political truth. It is that the *provisions and intentions of a given bill are not so important as the men [and women] who consider it and the atmosphere in which they function.*" (emphasis added)

Mills made an important addition to the legislation that was approved by the committee. The AMA's Eldercare plan would have extended the coverage under the Kerr-Mills Act to a broader range of seniors. Under Mills's plan, low-income seniors would not be the only ones to receive additional financial support for medical care. The Mills plan expanded this assistance to include the more than 3 million children under the age of 18 in families receiving cash welfare assistance under Aid to Families with Dependent Children (AFDC). It was also extended to the children's parents and to poor people who were blind or disabled. Referred to as Title XIX, this new program was estimated to cover up to 8 million people. The program was to be administered by state welfare departments. It was not mandatory, in that each state would have the option of adopting or electing not to adopt this new benefit.

After approval by the Ways and Means Committee, the legislation then went to the full House of Representatives for discussion and debate. On April 8, it was approved by a vote of 313-115, with 248 Democrats and 65 Republicans for and 73 Republicans and 42 Democrats against (Rosenblatt 2015, April 10).

After approval by the House, the bill then moved on to the Senate for consideration, where it came under the jurisdiction of the Finance Committee. An important member of the committee was Senator Russell Long of Louisiana. Long was a core member of the conservative southern block of senators—many of whom were still feeling the pain of the 1964 passage of the Civil Rights Act. On June 17, Senator Long succeeded in fundamentally altering the legislation in the committee from a hospital program for all elderly recipients of Social Security into another form of welfare that provided free hospital care only to the poor, with those with higher income paying a progressively larger share of the cost of their care.

Fortunately, the Senate Finance Committee reconsidered the amendments put forth by Long and on June 23, by a vote of 10-7, approved the original draft of the Medicare legislation. The committee then forwarded the legislation to the full Senate for consideration. President Johnson, as former Democratic majority leader in the Senate, was able to secure broad support. On July 9, the Senate passed the bill by a vote of 68-21; 55 Democrats and 13 Republicans voted for the legislation, while 7 Democrats and 14 Republicans voted against it. It is clear that

Medicare had achieved broad bipartisan backing both within Congress and in the country more generally (Rosenblatt 2015, July 10).

While the Senate passed the Medicare legislation by a wide margin, there were some core differences between it and the version passed by the House, which would need to be worked out in a House-Senate conference committee. The two versions differed over the length of the hospital care benefit, the proportion of patient payment for that care, the level of nursing home care provided, and patient eligibility for home health care. Both the House and the Senate bills agreed on what was referred to Medicare Part B, which covered payment for physician care. Enrollment in Part B would be voluntary and would involve a monthly premium. Part B would be administered by a private insurance company such as Blue Cross or Blue Shield, with federal reimbursement to these "fiscal intermediaries" for a majority of the cost of physician care. The House and Senate bills differed on the level of copayment for which patients would be responsible.

The conference committee addressed these and a long list of minor differences during a series of meetings held in mid-July. Given the strong bipartisan support for the "three-layer cake" legislation originally developed in the House Ways and Means Committee under the leadership of Wilbur Mills, the conference committee was able to work out the differences between the House and Senate versions of the legislation and send the final bill to the floor of both houses for final consideration. The final version of the bill was approved in the House on July 27 and in the Senate on July 28.

To honor President Truman's earlier efforts to institute national health insurance, President Johnson flew to Truman's home in Independence, Missouri, to sign the bill in his presence. Johnson signed the bill on July 30, thus enacting both Medicare and Medicaid as amendments to the preexisting Social Security Act. Medicare, referred to as Title XVIII, included two principal components:

1. Part A, which provided coverage of up to 90 days of hospital care during a spell of illness. The patient would pay the first $40 in costs and an additional $10 for each day of hospital care

over 60. Part A also covered up to 100 days of care in a nursing home for patients needing additional skilled care following a minimum 3-day hospital stay. Part A would be administered by the federal government and financed through a new payroll tax.

2. Part B, which was a new voluntary insurance program covering care provided by physicians. The program would be administered by private companies such as Blue Cross or Blue Shield. Patients would pay a small monthly premium (initially $3 per month) and would be free to receive care from any physician who had elected to participate in Medicare. Doctors would be free to charge what the law referred to as their "reasonable and customary charges." After meeting a yearly deductible, patients would pay 20% of the doctor's charge, and the private company acting as the intermediary would pay the remaining 80%. The company would then be reimbursed from general federal tax revenues for this amount.

As described by Marmor (1973, p. 80), "It was not required that the doctor directly charge the insurance company intermediaries who were to handle the government payments; he could bill the patient, who, after paying his debt, would be reimbursed by the insurance company." The law left it up to the doctor whether to bill the insurance intermediary or to bill the patient directly, with the patient assuming responsibility for filing the necessary paperwork with the intermediary.

Medicaid, referred to as Title XIX of the Social Security Act, would extend the funding provided to states under the Kerr-Mills Act of 1960. It expanded eligibility to seniors with incomes below a certain level as well as poor families with children who were receiving cash welfare benefits. Participation in Medicaid on the part of the states was strictly voluntary, and each state was left to decide on the maximum income and asset levels that would determine eligibility for coverage. The federal government would reimburse those states participating in the program for a defined share of the state's expenditure, with a higher rate of reimbursement for states with lower per-capita income.

Despite its earlier total opposition to the expansion of federal health care coverage, the AMA got the type of welfare-based coverage it had proposed under its Eldercare plan. An editorial published in the *New England Journal of Medicine* in August 1965 concluded that physicians essentially attained the outcome they had hoped for.

> Section VI of the A.M.A.'s *Principle of Ethics* states: "A physician should not dispose of his services under terms or conditions which tend to interfere with or impair the free and complete exercise of his medical judgment or tend to cause a deterioration of the quality of medical care." Those administering laws and regulations affecting a physician's practice should accept this principle, understand it and respect it—not as a concession to a reluctant participant in a federal program but because it is right and just and in the best interest of the patient, for whom the law was designed and to whom the physician is dedicated. (1965)

An article in *Science* from July 1965 reported on action taken by the AMA's House of Delegates in anticipation of the final passage of Medicare. Several state delegations proposed motions to encouraged doctors to boycott the new program. However, "the AMA leadership, sensitive to the loss of credibility and influence that its long isolation over medicare has already produced, came to New York opposing a boycott; a substantial portion of the delegates came to New York endorsing one; in the end, the leadership was victorious . . . when the emotional wave was spent, the move for a boycott was defeated" (Langer 1965, p. 166).

The Civil Rights Implications of Medicare and Medicaid

While the legislation enacting Medicare and Medicaid did not address the issue of civil rights and racial segregation directly, it had a powerful impact on the health care system as a consequence of components of the Civil Rights Act of 1964. To qualify for any federal payment under either Medicare or Medicaid, a hospital must comply with Title VI of the Civil Rights Act. As described by Surgeon General William H. Stewart (1966, p. 175), "Title VI prohibits discrimination on the basis of race, color, or national origin in any institution receiving financial aid from the US government . . . [T]hese guidelines spell out what discrimination is: when a patient, visitor, professional staff member, or trainee is treated differently solely because of his race, color, or national origin." Dr. Stewart went on to clarify what type of care would be expected: "Title VI does not require that there be a Negro and a white patient in every room, but it does require that all patients be assigned to rooms, wards, floors, or buildings of hospitals without regard to race, color, or national origin." In a similar manner, hospitals, principally in southern states, that refused to hire African American physicians were prohibited from participating in Medicare or Medicaid.

Although the AMA was the principal physicians' advocacy organization, for much of its history the AMA would not allow African American physicians to join the organization. In response, in 1895 Black doctors formed their own professional organization, the National Medical Association. In November 1966, Dr. Earl Belle Smith published an editorial in the *Journal of the National Medical Association* titled "Minorities and Medicare" voicing ardent support for it: "We maintain that the Medicare Law which provides hospital insurance and medical insurance will give the elderly minority a sense of dignity, self-attainment, equality, and much-needed justice" (1966, p. 466). Dr. Smith pointed out that it was not only hospitals in the South that had discriminated against African Americans in the provision of care (p. 467): "Historically that section of our country below the Mason-Dixon line which has been publicized and criticized as the forebearer of all aspects of discrimination and segregation in medical facilities and care for the Negro is not the singular citadel of medical bias in these fifty states. However, true records of history should profoundly proclaim that bigotry in medical care and medical practice has no geographical boundaries because these unjust practices exist in all sections of the United States."

In the same issue of the *Journal of the National Medical Association*, the Social Security commissioner reported on the success of Medicare in its first 60 days (Ball 1966, p. 475): "Currently 6,521 hospitals, accounting for 97 percent of the short-term general care hospital beds in the Nation, are participating in the program . . . We are still much concerned, however, about the situation in some communities in the South where between 200 and 250 hospitals have not yet taken the steps necessary to provide services on a nondiscriminatory basis." With millions of dollars of federal and state payment at stake, hospitals across the country eventually eliminated racial barriers to equal care within hospitals. "Ultimately, the desegregation of the health care facilities may create as much social change in this country as the provision of health care for tens of millions of seniors" (Rosenblatt 2015, July 30).

The National Reaction to Medicare

The benefits available to seniors under Medicare were due to go into effect on July 1, 1966. "Unprecedented efforts have also been made by the government to make sure that all of the country's more than 19 million elderly know about the program and understand why experts agree almost unanimously that it is a bargain" (Langer 1966, p. 1366). The federal government launched Operation Medicare Alert to get the word out to seniors, especially low-income seniors, to sign up for care. "Churches, scouts, civic groups, clubs—every conceivable source of manpower has been tapped for the campaign" (p. 1367). By March 8, 1966, 15 million seniors, comprising 79% of those eligible, had signed up. With seniors previously postponing needed medical treatment because of its cost, doctors and hospitals were bracing for a major surge in care.

In August 1966, Dr. Russell Roth, chairman of the AMA Council on Medical Services, published in *JAMA* a message to practicing physicians. "On balance, it is our feeling that the Social Security Administration, the Public Health Service, and the Secretary of Health, Education and Welfare with his staff have been receptive to our advice and have followed many, but clearly not all, of our recommendations" (Roth 1966, p. 125). In October 1966, the California Medical Association (CMA) reported in its journal on the success of the Medicare and the Medicaid program (Medi-Cal) in California: "California Physicians' Service and Occidental Life Insurance Company combined (two carriers in California administering Part B benefits) had received over three hundred thousand Medicare claims for physicians' services as of 30 September . . . The end of September marked the seventh complete month for the operation of the Medi-Cal program. The two Blue Cross Plans have processed over five hundred thousand claims from hospitals, nursing homes and home health agencies, and have paid over $100 million on these claims" (Wayburn 1966, pp. 305-6).

Dr. Edgar Wayburn, the editor of the CMA's journal, came to a seemingly positive assessment of these new federal programs that physicians had previously opposed so stridently. "The surprisingly smooth functioning of the programs thus far and the willingness of the administrative officers to give careful consideration to medical and hospital management suggestions for improvements in operation and equity, bespeak a mutual respect and spirit of cooperation that augur well for necessary changes and the preservation of good medical care to the eligibles" (p. 306).

Undersecretary of the U.S. Department of Health, Education and Welfare Cohen echoed Dr. Wayburn's assessment of Medicare's success in its first 100 days. "I think that it is safe to say that no single legislative act of the Federal Government will have a more beneficial effect upon the capacity of this country to provide high-quality health care to its citizens . . . The first 100 days of Medicare have been a truly remarkable achievement" (Cohen 1966, p. 1051). Cohen did acknowledge that "there is still cause for concern, however, about the situation in some communities in the South where between 150 and 200 facilities have not yet taken the steps necessary to provide services on a nondiscriminatory basis" (p. 1052).

Dr. Philip Bonnet, president of the American Hospital Association, while acknowledging that initially the AHA had resisted Medicare, following its passage concluded that "Medicare is another step forward—and a major one—on the long winding road with many ups and downs that had its beginning long ago" (1966, p. 995). Dr. Bonnet went on to suggest that the passage of Medicare had substantial historical significance (p. 996): "The development of the form that Medicare has acquired is *a fascinating case study of the operation and effectiveness of representative democratic government*. At the end, all the lessons that had been learned during the thirty years . . . were *woven by the magical arts of political compromise into an impressive tapestry*" (emphasis added).

TWO

Building on the Bipartisanship That Gained Passage of Medicare and Medicaid

AS WE saw in the closing of the previous chapter, the enactment in 1965 of Medicare and Medicaid "is a fascinating case study of the operation and effectiveness of representative democratic government . . . woven by the magical arts of political compromise into an impressive tapestry." However, we also saw at the beginning of the chapter that the process did not start out as a tapestry of political compromise. "It is difficult for many younger people today to realize how harsh many of the criticisms and arguments against these health proposals were" (Cohen 1985, p. 3).

When, in 1949, President Truman proposed a program of national health insurance, conservatives in Congress, both Democratic and Republican, joined the AMA in characterizing it as a first step toward socialized medicine in a form consistent with the theory of communism. In 2015 Julian Zelizer remarked in an article in the *New Yorker* marking the 50th anniversary of the passage of Medicare and Medicaid:

> When President Harry Truman proposed national health insurance for every American in 1945, and again in 1949, as part of his effort to move forward with domestic policies that had been left out of the New Deal,

he and allied liberals came to see why F.D.R. had avoided the issue of health care back in the nineteen-thirties . . . Charging that the Truman Administration consisted of "followers of the Moscow party line," the A.M.A. worked closely with the conservative coalition in Congress to kill the measure in committee. By 1950, the proposal was dead.

As a Republican, President Eisenhower also opposed any expansion of the Social Security program to include medical care. It was only in 1964, with substantial Democratic majorities in both the House and the Senate, that Wilbur Cohen and George Ball, working on behalf of President Johnson, won the support of Wilbur Mills, the powerful Democratic chairman of the House Ways and Means Committee, in crafting the "three-layer cake" compromise that created Medicare Parts A and B as well as Medicaid.

In 2015, 50 years later, our country again found itself deeply divided over the issue of health care—a divide deep enough to be considered a national chasm. In his 2015 history, Zelizer compares the enactment of Medicare and Medicaid to what we face as a country today: "But the passage of Medicare and Medicaid, which shattered the barriers that had separated the federal government and the health-care system, was no less contentious than the recent debates about the Affordable Care Act."

If the passage of Medicare and Medicaid represented a rare episode of bipartisanship and cross-party collaboration, what about the years coming after the beginning of these national health care programs? Did that bipartisanship persist? As we will see, over a period of more than thirty years, there continued to be collaboration and cooperation on these and other national health care issues.

Reforming How Hospitals Are Paid for the Care They Provide

During the tumultuous years of the Nixon presidency, followed by the short presidency of Gerald Ford, little action was taken to address national health care issues. In 1971, Nixon had proposed legislation creating an employer mandate to provide health insurance to employees, but Congress never acted on it.

In 1976, Jimmy Carter was elected president. During his campaign, he had often championed national health care reform. When he was inaugurated in January 1977, President Carter faced a more serious problem that commanded his attention: stagflation, a combination of falling GDP and rising prices. Rather than focus on national health care reform, President Carter instead focused his initial attention on rapidly rising hospital costs and the impact they were having on Medicare and Medicaid as well as the private market for health care.

Richard Lyons of the *New York Times* (1977) reported that, in April 1977, Carter sent Congress a proposal to impose cost controls on hospitals nationally as a first step in reining in rising health care expenditures. As described by the *CQ Almanac* (1977), "President Carter singled out hospital costs as the first target in his drive to put the brakes on skyrocketing health care costs in the United States." Under the proposed legislation, hospitals could increase the prices they charged for inpatient care by no more than 9% per year, with lower increases in subsequent years.

Legislation enacting President Carter's proposal was introduced in the House on April 25 as H.R. 6575. Ted Kennedy and two of his Democratic Senate colleagues introduced comparable legislation as S. 1391. Neither house of Congress took action on these bills during the 1977 legislative session. In 1978, the Senate passed a compromise bill, making the cost constraints voluntary. However, the House failed to take action, and it died with the end of the congressional session.

In the new session of Congress, President Carter resubmitted his proposal to Congress in March 1979, as H.R. 2626 and S. 570. Under the revised legislation, more than half of hospitals were granted exemptions from the price controls. Even so, the American Hospital Association and the American Medical Association mounted vigorous lobbying campaigns against it. In July, the House Ways and Means Committee approved a modified version of the bill. The House Commerce Committee passed it in September. In November, the full House voted it down 234-166. Members of both parties voted in opposition. Instead, by a bipartisan vote of 321-75, the House voted simply to create a national commission to study the issue of hospital costs. Members of both parties had collaborated to defeat Carter's hospital price controls.

Congress Defers to the Private Sector to Control Hospital Costs

Writing in 1978, former Social Security commissioner Robert Ball described some of the administrative and financial changes that had taken place in Medicare: "Medicare, by law and administrative regulation, has been shifting from the relatively passive role of insurer to taking an increasingly active role as a buyer of a defined product. The professional standards review organization (PSRO) requirement for a peer review of the necessity of service and the quality of care is perhaps the most notable example of the move toward product definition" (p. 866).

As described by White and Zimmerly (1974, p. 393), "PSRO is probably the most important health legislation ever enacted in the United States. Its capacity to improve quality of medical care is virtually unlimited." Under the PSRO legislation, physicians in each local community would select a group of qualified physicians who would have the authority to review the hospital care provided by their physician colleagues under Medicare or Medicaid to determine whether it met established quality standards. Substandard care might either be care that left out important steps or care that was unnecessarily costly.

I can recall an instance in the late 1970s when, as a practicing physician in a rural area of California, I had an elderly patient with unexplained abdominal pain. He lived by himself, with no family, up a long, winding dirt road on a mountainside. I made the decision to place the patient in the local community hospital to undertake a standard set of tests to diagnose and treat his condition. The day after I admitted the patient, I received a call from the physician chair of the hospital's PSRO committee. He suggested that it would have been more appropriate to conduct these tests on an outpatient basis. It was only after I explained the patient's unique living situation and my concern for his safety that the physician permitted me to keep the patient in the hospital, but only for a maximum of three days.

Although some physicians found the PSROs to be intrusive, by and large they were well regarded by physicians, as well as hospital administrators. This was a law implemented with bipartisan support. First introduced in the Senate Finance Committee by Wallace F. Bennett, a Republican from Utah, the law was passed in 1972. "Since Public Law 92-603 was enacted in October 1972 considerable progress has been made in the establishment of Professional Standards Review Organizations (PSROs) for the purpose of determining the necessity, appropriateness, and quality of medical care provided beneficiaries of the major programs authorized in the Social Security Act" (Ellis 1976, p. 370).

Notably, the same law that created PSROs also provided life-saving therapy. "Perhaps no other Federal Government program can lay claim to have saved as many lives as the Medicare end stage renal disease (ESRD) program. Since its inception in 1973, as a result of the Social Security Amendments of 1972 (Public Law 92-603, section 299I), over 1 million persons have received life-saving renal replacement therapy under this program" (Eggers 2000, p. 55).

Public Law 92-603 was passed by both houses of Congress on October 17, 1972. The vote in the House was 305-1. The vote in the Senate was 61-0 (Ball 1973), demonstrating wide bipartisan agreement that Medicare and Medicaid could be improved by changes in coverage and in quality review.

Throughout the 1970s, hospital expenditures under Medicare, which were paid out of the Medicare Hospital Insurance Trust Fund, continued to rise. The trust fund's sole source of financing was the payroll taxes created by the original Medicare legislation. Concerned about the stability of the trust fund, in 1981 President Reagan, by executive order, created the National Commission on Social Security Reform (NCSSR). The role of NCSSR was "to review the current and long-range financial condition of the Social Security trust funds and to report its findings and recommendations to the President and the Congress by December 31, 1982" (Svahn and Ross 1983, p. 6).

The original means of payment under Medicare was for the hospital to calculate the expenses involved in caring for a patient and then reporting those costs to Medicare. Medicare would then reimburse the hospital 100%, after subtracting the relatively small copayment the Medicare beneficiary was required to pay for each hospitalization. As one might imagine, there was little incentive for hospitals to hold down the costs of caring for Medicare patients. The more the hospital spent, the more it would receive as reimbursement.

President Reagan's NCSSR recommended a fundamental change in this means of hospital payment under Medicare: "The new law includes a major change in the method of payment under Medicare for inpatient hospital services. Effective with hospital cost-reporting periods beginning on or after October 1, 1983, for inpatient operating costs, Medicare will pay a fixed amount, determined in advance, for each case, according to one of 467 diagnosis-related groups (DRGs) into which a case is classified. The prospective payments will be considered payment in full" (Svahn and Ross 1983, p. 35). The DRGs established by the NCSSR were specific disease conditions, for example, a heart attack without serious complications. A heart attack with serious complications such as heart failure was a separate DRG category. Once the hospital had established the diagnosis for which the patient had been admitted and treated, Medicare would pay the hospital a predetermined fixed amount. This new system was referred to as the Prospective Payment System, as payment amounts were determined prospectively, in contrast to the previous system, which calculated hospital costs retrospectively after the treatment was completed.

The financial incentives were reversed from the previous system, which had incentivized hospitals to provide more care for each patient, to a system in which the hospital was incentivized to minimize both the length of stay and the resources used in treating the patient. Since the hospital received a fixed, prospectively determined payment based on the patient's diagnosis, the less care the hospital provided, the more money it was able keep once the costs of care were covered.

The NCSSR recognized that the Prospective Payment System created the incentive to reduce the amount of care provided to each patient, principally by discharging the patient sooner. To monitor the quality of the care hospitals provided under this new system, the NCSSR recommended a second major change to the quality review procedures mandated under Medicare—the creation of Peer Review Organizations (PRO).

A PRO was a private organization with staff trained in monitoring and evaluating the quality of care provided by hospitals, replacing the PSRO established by the 1972 Social Security amendments. "The specified functions of a PRO include reviewing: (a) the validity of diagnostic information provided by hospitals; (b) the completeness, adequacy, and quality of care provided; (c) the appropriateness of admissions and discharges; and (d) the appropriateness of care for which outlier payments are made" (Svahn and Ross 1983, p. 38). Any hospital that had not contracted with a private PRO to monitor the quality of the care it provided was ineligible for Medicare payments.

When Medicare was originally passed in 1965, the Johnson administration was explicit in stating that it was not their intent to have Medicare or any other federal agency control or manage the way in which medical care was provided. These assurances were repeatedly given to the AMA and to the AHA in an effort to earn their backing for Medicare. The shift to the Prospective Payment System for hospital payment and the mandatory monitoring by an independent PRO of the quality of care provided in the hospital were enormous administrative changes to the payment system under Medicare for these organizations to accept. President Reagan was, by historical standards, a fiscally conservative Republican. In the early 1960s, Reagan had distributed recordings of a speech he made criticizing Medicare as socialized medicine that threatened the independence of physicians and other providers. As president, Reagan strongly agreed with the recommendations of his National Commission on Social Security Reform for the shift to prospective payment and PROs.

Members in both the House and the Senate largely agreed with President Reagan and these recommendations of his commission. At the end of March 1983, the House passed the Social Security Amendments of 1983 (Public Law 98-21) by a vote of 243-102. Shortly after, the Senate passed the bill by a vote of 58-14. President Reagan signed the law on April 20, 1983. Nearly 20 years after the creation of Medicare, some of the most profound changes to the Medicare law, and from a policy perspective some of the most important, were approved with strong bipartisan support. The cooperation that enabled the creation of Medicare was persisting in the decades following.

The Bayh-Dole Act and Reform of Intellectual Property Rights for Scientific Discoveries

So far in this chapter I have addressed the role of bipartisanship in reforming administrative aspects of Medicare in the years after its initial passage. There was another legislative action that fundamentally changed the way scientific discoveries are translated into new medical treatments for the American public. This action was passed in 1980 with bipartisan support, although it was inconsistent over the course of the congressional approval process.

The law that accomplished these ends is Public Law 96-517, which amended existing US patent laws to add a new chapter titled "Chapter 38—Patent Rights in Inventions Made with Federal Assistance" (Patent and Trademark Law Amendments Act 1980). Section 200 states, "It is the policy and objective of the Congress to use the patent system to promote the utilization of inventions arising from federally supported research or development . . . to promote collaboration between commercial concerns and nonprofit organizations, including universities . . . to promote the commercialization and public availability of inventions made in the United States by United States industry and labor." This amendment to the patent laws is commonly known as the Bayh-Dole Act (US Department of Health and Human Services, n.d.).

In a history of the Bayh-Dole Act, Ashley Stevens, the director of the Office of Technology Transfer at Boston University, describes its major significance: "The Bayh-Dole Act of 1980 reversed 35 years of public policy and gave universities and small businesses the unfettered right to own inventions that resulted from federally funded research" (2004, p. 93). Based on its fundamental impact on the way patent rights are allocated for discoveries made with federal funding, an article in the journal the *Economist* (2002, p. 3) concluded, "Possibly the most inspired piece of legislation to be enacted in America over the past half century was the Bayh-Dole Act of 1980."

During the 1970s, a number of people both in Congress and in the Carter administration were concerned with the competitiveness of US businesses in a growing global economy. An issue that began to receive growing attention was the way the US government handled intellectual property rights to important discoveries made with federal funding. "Starting after World War II, the government had been taking an increasingly strident position that any inventions resulting from federally funded research belonged to the government and would only be non-exclusively licensed—the 'favor everyone one' philosophy" (Stevens 2004, p. 94). Specific offices within the Department of Health, Education and Welfare were given authority to grant universities that made important discoveries funded either in whole or in part by HEW the intellectual property rights to these discoveries. This authority was not available to other government departments or agencies.

In the 1970s, Purdue University made a series of important scientific discoveries with grant money from the US Department of Energy, which was not authorized to grant Purdue the intellectual property rights. Officials at Purdue went to Indiana senator Birch Bayh, a Democrat, and asked his help. Staff members from Senator Bayh's office approached the staff of his colleague Senator Robert Dole, Republican of Kansas.

Senators Bayh and Dole agreed that US patent law should be amended to assure universities of the intellectual property rights to any discoveries they made with federal funding. Their staffs worked collaboratively and submitted the first draft of the legislation to the Senate on September 13, 1978. The senators realized that they were unlikely to pass a bill submitted that late in a legislative session. Nonetheless, they shared the proposed legislation with their Senate colleagues to build momentum. They then reintroduced the bill in the new session of Congress convening in 1979. The Bayh-Dole bill was titled the University and Small Business Patent Procedures Act.

Beginning in May, the bill was the subject of hearings in the Senate Judiciary Committee. Elmer Staats, comptroller of the United States, testified that federal agencies' lack of authority to grant exclusive licensing rights to researchers discouraged broader investment by private companies in the economy. Interestingly, Admiral Hyman G. Rickover, a leader in the navy's development of nuclear-powered ships, argued against granting government-supported patent rights to private companies (Stevens 2004).

To address Rickover's concerns, Senators Bayh and Dole amended their bill to authorize the granting of patent rights only to universities and to small businesses. This change won the backing of a number of senators with major universities in their state, including important senators such as Ted Kennedy of Massachusetts, Strom Thurmond of South Carolina, and Gaylord Nelson of Wisconsin. On December 12, the Judiciary Committee unanimously approved the Bayh-Dole bill and sent it to the full Senate for consideration.

A key contributor to the success of Bayh-Dole was the wide support these two senators were able to cultivate among their senatorial colleagues. "A major reason for this support was that Senators Bayh and Dole were highly regarded in their respective parties and built political bridges between liberals and conservatives through their strong support of the measure" (Stevens 2004, p. 96). Following the tumultuous presidency of Richard Nixon, not only were senators and congressional representatives able to talk openly with their colleagues from the other party and those with differing political perspectives, they were also able to work collaboratively to find compromise approaches to issues of national import.

This ability of Senators Bayh and Dole to work collaboratively was essential, in light of differing perspectives some of their Senate colleagues held on the issue. Stevens identified Senators Adlai Stevenson, a Democrat from Illinois, and Harrison Schmitt, a Republican from New Mexico, as favoring the inclusion of large companies among those eligible for receiving intellectual property rights from government-funded research. By contrast, Senator Russell Long, a conservative from Louisiana, "was implacably opposed to big business getting ownership of government-funded patents" (Stevens 2004, p. 96). Long was also in the powerful position of chairman of the Senate Finance Committee.

Despite the opposition of these senators, when the Bayh-Dole bill came up for a final Senate vote on April 23, 1980, it was approved 91-4. Senators Bayh and Dole were clearly able to work together across party lines to achieve bipartisan enthusiasm for what some say is one of the most impactful laws of the twentieth century.

While the Senate was considering Bayh-Dole, the House of Representatives had been exploring an alternative bill sponsored by Representative Robert Kastenmeier, Democrat of Wisconsin and chair of the House Judiciary Committee. Kastenmeier's bill had the strong backing of the Carter administration for making large businesses eligible for patent rights. His bill was approved by the Judiciary Committee and sent to the House floor for discussion. The House failed to take final action on the Kastenmeier bill before it adjourned for the 1980 elections.

The outcome of this election had profound impacts on the direction the federal government was taking. Ronald Reagan defeated Jimmy Carter in the presidential election, and Republicans gained control of the Senate. Equally important, Birch Bayh was defeated in his reelection campaign. The outlook for the Bayh-Dole bill in the new Congress was bleak.

Following the November elections and before the new Congress took over, the current Congress needed to schedule a lame duck session to finalize the budget bills and other essential legislation that it had not finalized. Because the Bayh-Dole bill had not been discussed by the House, there was no clear road to passage during the brief session. There was, however, an alternative way to pass Bayh-Dole through bipartisan cooperation. Staff members from the Senate and the House Judiciary Committees got together and agreed to a compromise. Representative Kastenmeier's committee had passed a comprehensive omnibus patent bill that included large companies. There were equally important parts of the bill pertaining to other aspects of patent law that Kastenmeier wanted to push through but that faced potential opposition in the Senate. Representative Kastenmeier agreed to add the provisions of the Bayh-Dole bill to his legislation, in return for Bayh delivering Senate votes for the full patent bill.

The House quickly passed the combined bill. However, under the rules of a lame duck congressional session, every piece of legislation had to be passed by unanimous consent of both houses. Senator Russell Long had previously indicated his opposition to Bayh-Dole. All Long had to do was withhold his vote, and both Bayh-Dole and the omnibus patent bill would go down to defeat. However, he expressed a personal obligation to a long-standing Senate tradition—courtesy to other members under unique circumstances. In light of Senator Bayh's election defeat and imminent exit from the Senate, Long felt a duty to his colleague and added his vote to the unanimous Senate approval. The final version of the bill was sent to President Carter for his signature.

President Carter was also a lame duck. He had only 10 days to sign the legislation sent to him by Congress. If he withheld his signature, it would not become law, as there would be no opportunity for Congress to override a formal veto, what is often referred to as a "pocket veto." The senior staff of Bayh's Senate committee conveyed to White House staff the implications of failing to sign the bill in light of Senator Bayh's imminent departure. On December 12, 1980, President Carter signed the bill, and the Bayh-Dole Act became law. To this day, universities and small, mostly nonprofit companies that make major scientific discoveries with federal grant funding are able to take ownership of the patent rights to their discovery and to license those rights to private pharmaceutical companies and other for-profit entities, receiving millions of dollars in royalties in return. A report by Pressman and colleagues (2015) estimates that, between 1996 and 2013, academic licensing of scientific discoveries added as much as $1.18 trillion to industry economic output.

The Bayh-Dole Act fundamentally changed university/industry relations. Although not all scholars or policy analysts agree that this arrangement is still in the best interest of the country, the law continues to have major economic and academic impacts. As Stevens concludes in his history of the Bayh-Dole Act (2004, p. 97), "The U.S. Senate is rightly proud of its tradition of Senatorial courtesy, and Long's willingness to yield on an issue on which he felt so strongly is a stunning example of this courtesy. It is hard to imagine an act of such Senatorial courtesy in the current climate in Congress."

Stevens wrote these words in 2004. It is even harder to imagine an act of such senatorial courtesy in the divisive political atmosphere confronting our country today. As I will suggest at the end of this book, however, I truly believe that it is possible, given the right people and the right incentives, to recover such courtesy again.

Bipartisanship Stumbles with the Clintons' Health Security Act

By the end of the 1980s, national health insurance was back on the American political agenda. In 1989, the *New England Journal of Medicine* published a series of articles proposing major reforms to the American health care system with the goal of providing universal coverage. The first proposal was published as a series of two articles by Alain Enthoven and Richard Kronick (1989a, 1989b). The authors described a new way of providing health insurance under which "everyone not covered by an existing public program would be enabled to buy affordable subsidized coverage, either through their employers, in the case of full-time employees, or through 'public sponsors,' in the case of the self-employed and all others." Under their proposal, "the federal government would enact legislation giving each state powerful incentives to create a 'public sponsor' agency to act as sponsor for people otherwise unsponsored" (1989a, p. 31). A public sponsor would be a nonprofit broker that provides a series of health insurance options offered by private insurance companies. Individuals who lack health insurance could then select from among these plans based on the relative price of each plan and the quality of the care they offer. The sponsor would monitor the quality of the care provided by each of the plans included in its list of options.

The authors went on to describe what they perceived as the characteristics any plan for a new approach to universal health insurance requires for the public as well as political acceptance. "Such a plan must represent incremental, not radical, change; must respect the preferences of voters, patients, and providers; must avoid major disruption in satisfactory existing arrangements; must avoid creating major windfall gains or losses; must avoid large-scale income redistribution; and must not be inflationary" (Enthoven and Kronick 1989b, p. 94). In a later publication, Enthoven (1993) would describe his plan as "managed competition." This became the model on which the Clinton administration forged its own proposal for national health insurance.

In the same issue of the *New England Journal of Medicine* that contained the second part of the Enthoven and Kronick proposals, David Himmelstein and Steffie Woolhandler (1989, p. 102) presented their vision for national health insurance: "We envisage a program that would be federally mandated and ultimately funded by the federal government but administered largely at the state and local level . . . Our plan borrows many features from the Canadian national health program and adapts them to the unique circumstances of the United States." Modeled on the Canadian system, the authors indicate that their plan would establish a "single payer for services" and "overall [national] spending limits."

In the same year that Enthoven and Kronick and Himmelstein and Woolhandler published their proposals for national health insurance, Senator Ted Kennedy, chair of the Labor and Human Resources Committee, and Senator Don Riegle, chair of the Finance Committee's Subcommittee on Health for Families and the Uninsured, created a bi-committee bipartisan Senate Working Group on Universal Access (Peterson 1992). Following meetings held over a period of six months, the working group was replaced by a bipartisan steering committee, which included Democratic senators Riegle and Kennedy as well as Republican senators John Chafee and Orrin Hatch.

By December 1990, the steering committee drafted a series of proposals, with Democrats favoring an employer mandate to cover all workers and Republicans calling for an expansion of public programs to cover uninsured individuals. "Ultimately, however, the process disintegrated, apparently when Senator Hatch would not yield at all in his objections to the various proposed mandates or incentives to compel employers to provide health insurance benefits to their workers" (Peterson 1992, p. 557). The bipartisan effort had come close to an agreement but in the end failed.

In 1991, Robert Blendon and Jennifer Edwards of Harvard University reported that a growing number of Americans favored the concept of universal health insurance coverage. Based on polling data, they reported that 72% of the general public, 67% of corporate executives, and 92% of labor union leaders called for adopting universal health insurance coverage, "even if it means an increase in taxes" (p. 2563).

In April 1991, Senator John Heinz, a Republican from Pennsylvania, was killed in a plane crash. Democrat Harris Wofford was appointed to fill Heinz's seat, pending a special election to be held in November 1991. In that election, Wofford ran against former Pennsylvania governor and former US attorney general Richard Thornburgh. Preelection polls showed Wofford trailing 45 points behind Thornburgh.

Wofford chose to focus his campaign on the need for national health insurance. Polls showed a similar level of support among Pennsylvania voters for the adoption of national health insurance as the national polls cited by Blendon and Edwards: "75 percent of the public favored (and 50 percent strongly favored) 'creating a system of national health insurance,' and 63 percent were more likely to vote for the candidate who favored such a program" (Peterson 1992, p. 570).

As reported in the *New York Times* (Hinds 1991), "In a stunning upset that will raise the hopes of Democrats and the fears of Republicans facing elections next year, Harris Wofford, a little-known Democrat with an anti-Bush message, today trounced former Attorney General Dick Thornburgh . . . With 87 percent of 9,428 precincts reporting, the vote was: Wofford 1,594,443 (56 percent), Thornburgh 1,270,355 (44 percent)." Peterson describes the impact of this election (1992, p. 570): "First, Wofford became a symbol to the Democrats of what they could achieve in the 1992 election, both in Congress and for the presidency. Second, after the end of the first session, House and Senate Democratic leaders engaged in more intensive joint deliberations about how to formulate parallel leadership initiatives in both houses of Congress."

In an editorial published in May 1992, George D. Lundberg, the editor of *JAMA*, suggested that recent political activity and shifting public attitudes "have brought health care reform to the forefront of the US national agenda" (p. 2521). Lundberg argued, "In successful health care reform, all players and all stakeholders will have to compromise—the patients, the physicians, the insurance companies, the hospitals, the government, the politicians, and all the special interest groups. But the essence of compromise means that the major players all give up something and get something" (p. 2524).

In that same issue, Blendon, Edwards, and Hyams (1992) reviewed a series of 20 proposals for different types of health care reform submitted by members of Congress in 1991. They also referenced the AMA's proposal for national health insurance (Todd et al. 1991) and described the core aspects of those designed by each of the four leading candidates for president in the November 1992 elections: George H. W. Bush, Bill Clinton, Bob Kerry, and Paul Tsongas.

During the presidential campaign, Bill Clinton enlisted the assistance of a group of experienced health policy analysts, including Paul Starr and Walter Zelman. "Building upon and modifying ideas from economist Alain Enthoven . . . these advisers convinced Clinton that it would be possible to use regional insurance purchasing agencies along with modest new tax subsidies to push the employer-based U.S. health care system toward cost efficiency and universal coverage" (Skocpol 1995, p. 69). In 1991, Enthoven and Kronick published an updated version of the plan they had published in the *New England Journal of Medicine*. Following the advice of Zelman, Starr, and other advisors who had joined his campaign, Clinton campaigned on establishing a national health care program that relied on "competition within a budget."

The 1992 presidential election had three major candidates: George H. W. Bush, Bill Clinton, and Ross Perot, running as an Independent. Clinton received 43% of the popular vote, Bush received 37%, and Perot received 19%. Despite drawing only a plurality of the popular vote, Clinton won 370 electoral votes, out of a total of 538.

One of the first tasks President-Elect Clinton did was to convene a formal Health Reform Task Force. He asked his business colleague and friend Ira Magaziner and First Lady Hillary Rodham Clinton to lead the task force. The task force began by consulting with "hundreds of government officials, health policy experts, congressional staffers, and some state-level officials" (Skocpol 1995, p. 70).

In 1993, Starr and Zelman, as leading members of the task force, published a detailed description of their plan. They summarized the Clinton plan as based on the concept of managed competition put forth by Enthoven and Kronick. "The central innovation is the development of regional health insurance purchasing cooperatives (HIPCs) as managers and reorganizers of the market and platforms for global budgets" (p. 8). The HIPC was the new name given to the public sponsor described in Enthoven and Kronick's earlier work.

In the introduction to their article, Starr and Zelman write (1993, p. 8), "In some minds the word compromise raises the specter of compromised principles and corrupt bargains. But in a democracy compromise is not merely unavoidable; it is a source of creative invention, sometimes generating solutions that unexpectedly combine seemingly opposed ideas." Before describing the specifics of their plan, they ask, "Can our politics produce a strong compromise to restructure the system, extend insurance to all, and bring costs under control?"

The authors describe their plan, referred to as the Health Security Plan, as offering something both to conservatives and to liberals. It would be the job of the HIPC to "contract with varied private health plans, including health maintenance organizations (HMOs), preferred provider organizations (PPOs), and one free-choice-of-provider option. The plans would be paid by capitation," a fixed per-member per-month payment (Starr and Zelman 1993, p. 10). All Americans, including employees of small and midsized firms, would be able to go to the HIPC to select a plan. Employers with 1,000 employees or more would be free to establish their own HIPC. For people with full-time jobs, the employer would pay most of the cost of the health insurance plan selected by the employee, who would pay the balance. Those workers selecting a more expensive plan would pay a larger share of the premium. Those who were unemployed or employed only part time would receive a government subsidy to help them purchase a plan.

The task force charged by President Clinton with working out the details of his Health Security Plan began its work in earnest immediately after his inauguration in January 1993. Paul Starr has described some of the challenges the task force faced: "On the political calendar, health care first gave way to other priorities. During the presidential transition and his initial year in office, Clinton concentrated on the economy and the budget. The battle of the budget dragged on into the summer of 1993 and threatened his presidency; he had little choice but to focus on winning it" (1995).

It took the task force until the early summer of 1993 to commit a draft of their health care reform plan to paper. While Starr and Zelman had published a general description of the plan in early 1993, the task force kept the details of the proposal confidential. President Clinton finally introduced his Health Security Act in a speech to Congress on September 22, 1993. When the legislation worked out by the task force was submitted to Congress, it was 1,342 pages long (Skocpol 1995, p. 72).

In her 1995 article "The Rise and Resounding Demise of the Clinton Plan," Theda Skocpol chronicled (p. 67):

> The night of 22 September 1993 President Bill Clinton gave a stirring speech to Congress and the nation, calling for "America to fix a health care system that is badly broken . . . giving every American health security . . . Millions listened to the president, and polls taken right after the speech and over the next few weeks registered strong support.
>
> How ironic, then, that just barely a year later both the Clinton plan and the Democratic party—the legatee of the New Deal whose achievements President Clinton had hoped to imitate and extend—lay in a shambles.

Despite the months of work the members of the task force had put into crafting the Health Security Act, it never attracted the support in either the House or the Senate necessary for approval.

Paul Starr (1995), in his article titled "What Happened to Health Care Reform?," described what it felt like to be a leader of the task force that developed the Health Security Act, only to see it go down to defeat. "It was one year from euphoria to defeat . . . At first it seemed Clinton would move the country . . . A year later, almost to the day, Senate Majority Leader George Mitchell pronounced health care reform dead." Starr went on to recount his understanding of why the Health Security Act came up short:

The collapse of health care reform in the first two years of the Clinton administration will go down as one of the great lost political opportunities in American history. It is a story of compromises that never happened, of deals that were never closed . . . It is also a story of strategic miscalculation on the part of the president and those of us who advised him . . . Overconfident about the momentum of reform, we misjudged the health care politics of 1993 as a change in the climate when it was only a change in the weather.

Later in his discussion of why the Clinton act failed, Starr made another crucial point: "Perhaps the fateful choice was the decision to design a proposal inside the White House and put the Clinton name on it . . . The real problem was that time was spent developing a plan that should have been spent negotiating it."

The history of the passage of Medicare and Medicaid in 1965 underscores the essential role leaders in Congress play in negotiating a compromise that meets the needs and expectations of various factions. That lesson appears to have been lost on President Clinton and his task force. As an additional complexity, Starr concluded that "the First Lady's role further muddied the issue."

One of the central components of the proposal was the creation of more than 50 "health alliances" nationally to act as HIPCs for both individuals and small to medium-sized employers in selecting among competing health plans. The public perception of these alliances was of a massive new government bureaucracy charged with regulating health care. The continued success of small to midsized health insurance companies was threatened by these purchasing cooperatives. Collectively, these companies sponsored a series of national advertisements known as the "Harry and Louise" ads. These ads portrayed a white, seemingly middle-class couple who were afraid that the Clinton plan would take away their health insurance. At the conclusion of the ads, Louise would turn to Harry and say, "Harry, there must be a better way." (Several of these ads are available on YouTube for viewing.)

The complexity of the legislation, the process of delivering to Congress a final draft of the legislation created without congressional input, and the timing of the 1994 elections all contributed the defeat of Clinton's Health Security Act. In Starr's closing words (1995), "The lesson for next time in health reform is faster, smaller. We made the error of trying to do too much at once, took too long, and ended up achieving nothing."

In concluding her analysis of why the Health Security Act failed, Skocpol (1995, p. 81) speaks with a more optimistic voice. "Health reformers searching for optimistic historical analogies often take heart in the example of President Harry S. Truman. After his campaign for universal health insurance was defeated in 1948–1950, Truman and his allies devised an 'incremental' strategy that eventually led to the enactment of Medicare in 1965. Reformers dream of doing this again, perhaps pushing toward universal health insurance by next focusing on extending coverage to all American children." By 1997, Skocpol's optimism proved to be well warranted.

Expanding Health Insurance for Children through Bipartisan Collaboration

When Medicaid was first established in 1965, it provided medical care to families with young children who had previously qualified for cash welfare assistance under the Aid to Families with Dependent Children (AFDC) program. Under AFDC, each state sets the maximum level of income a family may earn and still qualify for cash assistance. States also define the family structure eligible for AFDC, with most limiting it to single-parent families. By 1978, the income cutoffs varied widely: for a family with one adult and three children, the maximum permissible monthly income varied from $187 in Texas to $560 in Vermont (Chief 1979, p. 20). In more than half of states, the maximum permissible income for a family of four was less than $350. In 1978, the federal poverty level for such a family was $6,200 per year (US Bureau of Labor Statistics 1979). This translates to a monthly income of $517. Only three states (Hawaii, Vermont, and Wisconsin) covered all families under the poverty line. The average income limit among the 50 states and the District of Columbia was $343, roughly two-thirds of the national poverty level. Eleven of the states had income limits that were less than 50% of the poverty level.

As increasing numbers of poor children went without health insurance because of the state variation in eligibility levels, finding a way to provide coverage for these children became an increasingly important policy goal. As Mann, Rowland, and Garfield describe in their "Historical Overview of Children's Health Care Coverage" (2003, p. 32), "For the past two decades, however, broad, consistent political support for health coverage for children has extended publicly funded coverage for children well beyond traditional welfare populations."

Increasing national attention to the health care needs of children was triggered by congressional approval under the Reagan administration of the Omnibus Budget Reconciliation Act of 1981 (OBRA). "OBRA mandated reductions in the federal match to states for a three-year period. In addition, it modified provisions of the 'work incentive' program within the AFDC program. As a result, an estimated 442,000 working poor families were eliminated from Medicaid" (Oberg and Polich 1988, p. 87). By 1985, 11 million children were without health insurance. "This disproportionate representation of children is due in large part to the wide variability in AFDC eligibility from state to state. The ten states with the lowest AFDC income levels cover only 38 percent of their children living below the poverty threshold. An aggregate national percentage has Medicaid covering less than half of the poor children in this country" (p. 90).

Responding to data such as these, Congress passed a series of laws over the following decade that increased access to health insurance coverage under Medicaid to children in poor families (Mann, Rowland, and Garfield 2003, pp. 34–35):

- The Deficit Reduction Act of 1984, which "required coverage for children born after September 30, 1983, up to age five, in families meeting state AFDC income and resource standards" (approximately 40% of the federal poverty level)
- The Omnibus Reconciliation Act of 1986, which allowed states to cover pregnant women and young children up to age 5 in

families with incomes at or below 100% of the federal poverty level

- The Omnibus Reconciliation Act of 1987, which allowed states to cover pregnant women and infants with family incomes at or below 185% of the federal poverty level, required coverage for children up to age 8 with family incomes below AFDC standards, and allowed states to cover these children up to 100% of the federal poverty level
- The Family Support Act of 1988, which required Medicaid coverage of two-parent families meeting the AFDC eligibility test with incomes below AFDC income, even if the state did not cover such families under AFDC
- The Omnibus Budget Reconciliation Act of 1989, which required coverage of pregnant women and children under age 6 in families with incomes at or below 133% of the federal poverty level
- The Omnibus Budget Reconciliation Act of 1990, which phased in (by 2002) coverage of all children ages 6–18 in families with incomes at or below 100% of the federal poverty level.

By the time Bill Clinton was elected president in 1992, Medicaid was in the process of expanding coverage to all children in the country whose families fell under the poverty level, that is, all poor children. Had Clinton's Health Security Act been approved by Congress, all children in the United States would have been eligible for health insurance coverage. Considering the failure of the act, broad bipartisan support for finding a way to extend health insurance coverage for America's children persisted.

A first step in reaching this goal was the passage in 1996 of the Personal Responsibility and Work Opportunity Reconciliation Act, which replaced the AFDC welfare program with Temporary Assistance for Needy Families (TANF). Under TANF, the link between the receipt of welfare benefits and eligibility for Medicaid was severed. With Medicaid coverage expanding to all children in families living below the poverty line, increasing national attention began to focus on children living in "near-poor" families, typically defined as those families with incomes between 100% and 200% of FPL.

The Medicaid law gave states the option of extending eligibility to children in near-poor families while receiving federal matching funds for them. By 1997, fewer than one-third of states had elected to expand coverage to these children. In Congress, there was disagreement regarding how best to extend coverage to them. "Some advocated expanding Medicaid to cover more low-income children, while others advocated a federal block grant that would give states virtually unlimited flexibility. The result was a compromise approach and the enactment in 1997 of SCHIP" (Mann, Rowland, and Garfield 2003, p. 38).

The State Children's Health Insurance Program was introduced in Congress in 1997. "The design of SCHIP reflects the fact that the legislation was the product of a political compromise between those advocating for a new health care block grant with little or no federal standards and those who supported a new Medicaid expansion for children" (Mann, Rowland, and Garfield 2003, p. 38). Under SCHIP, each state was eligible for a fixed block grant to finance the provision of health insurance to children in families between 100% and 200% of the FPL. States were required to pay a percentage of the cost of the program, but the states' cost-sharing requirement was substantially below that required under Medicaid coverage. States also had flexibility. "The design of the coverage expansion allows states three options for structuring their programs: They may use their federal SCHIP funds to create or expand a separate child health program, expand Medicaid, or use a combination of both types of programs." Given that the federal funds were provided through a fixed block grant, states had the option of freezing enrollment of eligible children in any year in which expenditures would exceed the funding provided by the block grant.

In the House of Representatives, the SCHIP legislation was reviewed by the Commerce Committee, which voted 39-7 in favor. In the Senate, the legislation was reviewed by the Finance Committee, which voted 20-0 to approve SCHIP. Differences between the two bills were settled in a conference committee. The revised legislation was then sent to both chambers, where it was approved in the House by a vote of 346-85 and in the Senate by a vote of 85-15 (*CQ Almanac* 1997).

Oberlander and Lyons (2009, p. w400) have described the success of SCHIP in these terms: "SCHIP rose from the ashes of the Clinton administration's failed Health Security Act. Congressional leaders had scarcely pronounced the Clinton plan dead in September 1994 when proposals to expand health insurance for low-income children emerged . . . SCHIP became law 'in record time' largely because it was everything the 1993 Clinton health reform plan was not."

Bipartisanship Stumbles Again under George W. Bush

When Medicare was passed in 1965, one important benefit was left out: coverage of prescription drugs. Medicare paid for prescription medications administered directly in either a hospital or a physician's office but provided no coverage for prescriptions for seniors to take on their own. With seniors facing rising financial strain due to the cost of prescription drugs, Congress made repeated attempts to extend Medicare coverage to include these expenses.

With the backing of both Republicans and Democrats, Congress did include prescription drug coverage when it passed the Medicare Catastrophic Coverage Act (MCCA) of 1988, President Reagan's last year in office. It was passed with substantial bipartisan majorities in both houses of Congress: by a vote of 328-72 in the House and 86-11 in the Senate (*CQ Almanac* 1988). It was only after passage of MCCA that seniors realized that the prescription drug coverage it provided was to be paid for by a highly progressive tax on seniors themselves. "The progressive financing proved to be the Achilles' heel of the MCCA, however. It meant that one-third of the elderly population—those with higher incomes—would be paying for more than two-thirds of the cost of the new benefits" (Oliver, Lee, and Lipton 2004, p. 299). When word of these new taxes got to the organizations representing seniors, they mobilized a strong opposition to the new law. "A public campaign for repeal of the MCCA was led by the National Committee to Preserve Social Security and Medicare, joined by a 40-group coalition of unions and other groups and several grassroots organizations" (p. 300). In November 1989, Congress took action to repeal the new prescription drug coverage as well as other provisions in the law.

The subsequent failure of the Clinton administration to pass the Health Security Act left prescription drug coverage for seniors in a very difficult position. The shift in congressional leadership following the election of 1994 was to have a major impact on subsequent bipartisan efforts. "The ideological shift in the Republican Party, which was first manifested in the 1970s and became more dramatic after the 1994 congressional elections, has transformed much of Medicare policymaking from a deliberative, bipartisan process into a highly polarized, deadlocked debate" (Oliver, Lee, and Lipton 2004, p. 289).

The Balanced Budget Act of 1997, which authorized SCHIP, also created a new program, Medicare Part C, or "Medicare + Choice." Under Part C, Medicare beneficiaries were given the option of enrolling in HMOs or PPOs as an alternative to the traditional, fee-for-service Medicare under Parts A and B. It set a yearly payment rate for these new delivery options that was several percentage points lower than the comparable costs under traditional Medicare. As a consequence, several of these managed care providers elected to drop out of Medicare, rather than face lower payments.

When George W. Bush was elected in 2000, after the extremely contentious *Bush v. Gore* controversy about the final vote in Florida, he made the decision to try to woo these private, market-based alternative systems back into Medicare. In setting this goal early in his administration, he also elected to include a new form of private, market-based prescription drug coverage as an option for Medicare beneficiaries. Republican leaders in the House and Senate submitted "a series of proposals to include a prescription drug benefit as essentially an inducement for beneficiaries to shift from the traditional fee-for-service program to a private health plan" (Oliver, Lee, and Lipton 2004, p. 306).

Democrats also favored a new prescription drug benefit as a component of Medicare, to be administered by the federal government. As a result of the 2002 elections, Republicans gained a majority in both the House and the Senate. Having perhaps learned a lesson from President

Clinton's failure to pass the Health Security Act, rather than submit proposed legislation himself, President Bush provided leaders of the House and Senate with a general description of the programs he would like to see and left it to Congress to write the actual legislation. This strategy seemed to work. By June 2003, the Senate Finance Committee had drafted a bipartisan agreement, which was then introduced as Senate Bill 1, the Prescription Drug and Medicare Improvement Act. The full committee approved the bill by a vote of 16-5.

Consistent with the guidance offered by President Bush, the bill included a maximum 10-year budget of $400 billion to pay for prescription drug coverage for Medicare beneficiaries. The new coverage would be available to seniors in one of two ways: either by joining one of the new Medicare managed care options created under the Balanced Budget Act of 1997 or by remaining in traditional Medicare and enrolling in a new, private-market prescription drug plan. Medicare itself would have no role in providing the coverage.

The bipartisanship displayed by the Finance Committee was replicated in the full Senate, which passed the bill on June 27 by a vote of 76-21. It was introduced in the House as H.R. 1, where it was considered by both the Ways and Means Committee and the Energy and Commerce Committee. Ways and Means passed the bill by a vote of 25-15. The legislation underscored the fact that the new prescription drug coverage would be available only through private market organizations, with no role for Medicare.

The House bill also included a formal prohibition against Medicare playing any role in setting drug prices, including direct negotiations with pharmaceutical companies. Democrats in the House responded strongly to these prohibitions and mounted an organized opposition to the bill. Nevertheless, the bill passed the House by a vote of 216-215. To reach this majority, the Bush administration had to reassure congressional Republicans that the 10-year cost of the new program would not exceed $400 billion. Republicans also wanted the bill to include stronger measures to encourage Medicare beneficiaries to shift from traditional Medicare into a private-market option. In part to assuage these Republicans, the bill also included additional funding to increase the amount

Medicare would pay private managed care plans to a level substantially above what it would otherwise have cost Medicare to provide comparable coverage under the traditional plans. This addition made Democratic opposition even stronger.

Given the close vote in the House, the Republican leadership heavily stacked membership in the House-Senate conference committee with Republicans who were behind the bill. As a result, it took four months for the committee to come up with the combined legislation. On November 15, it submitted the Medicare Prescription Drug, Improvement, and Modernization Act of 2003 to both houses for a final review and vote.

On November 17, much to the surprise of many in Congress, the American Association of Retired Persons (AARP) announced its endorsement of the legislation. After hours of discussion and debate, at 3:00 a.m. on November 22, the House passed the bill by a vote of 220-215, but only after President Bush personally called several Republican members and asked them to switch their votes. Only 16 Democrats supported the bill, while 25 Republicans voted in opposition. In the Senate, the final vote was 54-44 in for the bill, with 9 Republicans against and 11 Democrats and 1 independent in favor.

In January 2004, the president's Office of Management and Budget announced that it had revised the projected cost of the new prescription drug coverage to $534 billion over 10 years, substantially above the $400 billion estimate the legislation had included. "In March 2004 the chief actuary of the Centers for Medicare & Medicaid Services revealed that as early as the previous summer, his office had estimated much higher costs for the proposed reforms than congressional budget analysts had. His superiors in the Bush administration, however, ordered him to withhold the estimates from members of Congress and warned him that 'the consequences for insubordination [would be] extremely severe'" (Oliver, Lee, and Lipton 2004, p. 323). Whatever sense of bipartisanship had existed in Congress when it first started discussing President Bush's proposal for prescription drug coverage largely dissipated, with substantial resentment within both parties when the previously hidden cost estimates were revealed.

The CHIP on Bush's Shoulder Leads to a Schism

As described earlier in this chapter, SCHIP, the health insurance program for children in families earning between 100% and 200% of the FPL, became law "in record time" because of wide popularity across party lines. As Oberlander and Lyons (2009, p. w401) concluded, "SCHIP passed because it embraced the politics of compromise." By 2007, more than 6 million children were covered by SCHIP.

The original legislation authorizing SCHIP provided 10 years of funding. Accordingly, in 2007, Congress needed to reauthorize this funding to maintain the program. SCHIP had permitted states to provide health insurance to children in families earning up to 200% of the FPL. Under certain circumstances, some states were authorized to cover children up to 250% of poverty. By 1997, 26 states were covering children up to 200%, while 15 states were covering children above 250%. Nine states covered only children in families earning less than 200% of FPL (*CQ Almanac* 2007).

In the 2006 elections, Democrats won majorities in both the House and Senate, something that had not occurred since 1994. Based on the widespread success of SCHIP, as well as rising costs of health insurance that put substantial strains on working families, Democrats wanted to extend SCHIP funding for an additional 10 years and to expand the eligibility level to include families making up to 300% of the FPL. The estimated $35 billion in additional costs to provide this coverage would come from a new tobacco tax. In August 2007, the Senate passed the SCHIP reauthorization by a vote of 68-31. The House bill would have reauthorized SCHIP funding, as well as reduced some of the additional funding the 2003 Medicare Modernization Act had provided to encourage private managed care plans to participate. This triggered some opposition among Republicans, but the House nevertheless passed the combined legislation by a vote of 225-204.

Democrats and Republicans held a series of negotiations to reconcile the differences between the House and Senate versions of the bill. The compromise the parties reached largely accepted the Senate version of the bill. This led to a vote in favor of the compromise bill of 265-159 in the House and 67-29 in the Senate. Under the compromise, eligibility for SCHIP was capped at 300% of FPL. It also included the potential for individual states to request a waiver to cover children in families up to 400%.

When President Bush learned of the compromise, he spoke at a news conference and announced that he planned to veto the bill. He was stridently opposed to expanding SCHIP eligibility for families with incomes above 200% of FPL. Bush "said that it would 'move millions of American children who now have private health insurance into government-run health care' and would raise taxes on 'working people.' The plan, he said, would turn a program meant to help poor children into 'one that covers children in households with incomes of up to $83,000 a year'" (*CQ Almanac* 2007). Bush vetoed the bill on October 3. On October 18, the House voted 273-156 to override the president's veto—13 votes short of the two-thirds majority required.

Democrats in the House and Senate rapidly came up with a revised bill that put a firm cap of 300% of the FPL for eligibility. Democrats in the House expedited the committee hearing process and brought the bill to the floor on October 25 for a final vote. The House approved 265-142. The bill moved to the Senate, where it was passed on November 1 by a vote of 64-30. On December 12, President Bush vetoed the bill for a second time.

When Congress reconvened after the holiday break, the House once again attempted to override President Bush's veto. Again the motion to overturn failed, this time by a vote of 260-152. Fortunately, earlier in the session, Congress had approved and President Bush had signed a temporary measure to keep the original SCHIP funded through March 2009.

From the time Congress first approved SCHIP during the Clinton administration, there was strong cross-party unity to provide children in low income, working families with taxpayer-funded health insurance. That unity among Democrats and Republicans continued into the Bush administration. Bipartisan majorities in both the House and the Senate approved an extension of SCHIP, broadening the number of children who would be eligible for care.

Bush, however, had strong opposing views. Rather than attempting to work with the congressional leaders of both parties, he refused even to discuss the full renewal of SCHIP. "The Bush administration's opposition to SCHIP expansion was largely ideological. Administration officials argued that SCHIP expansion would push the U.S. toward 'a single-payer health care system with rationing and price controls.' President Bush labeled SCHIP expansion a step 'down the path to government-run health care for every American.' The administration apparently saw SCHIP as a front in a broader ideological struggle over health reform, and it was unwilling to give any ground" (Oberlander and Lyons 2009, p. w405). The Bush vetoes and the schism they created were to become a major issue in the political discussions leading up to the 2008 elections.

THREE

Health Care Reform under the
Obama Administration

Health Care Reform and the 2008 Elections

By June 2008, it was becoming increasingly clear to the American public who the major party nominees for president would be. John McCain had received the pledges of more than enough convention delegates to be the presumptive nominee. Barack Obama had won more than enough delegates through the primary elections to assure him the nomination, leading Hillary Clinton to announce later that she was suspending her campaign and endorsing Obama for president.

With their nominations virtually assured, the public discussion turned to the issue at the top of the political agenda: health care. An editorial in the *Lancet* (2008a, p. 1971) published shortly afterward reported, "For many Americans, especially the large number of uninsured and underinsured, the most pressing domestic concern is health care." By that time, both candidates had broadly outlined their approach to national health care reform. The editorial went on to describe the principal focus of each candidate's plan: "In traditional Republican style, McCain believes in market-based solutions to health-care reform. He would not dismantle the employer-based insurance system, but would provide tax credits to make it more affordable . . . Obama's plan is also predictably Democratic, although it is not as radical as the single-payer plan favoured by the most liberal wing of the party. His plan instead is a compromise of sorts."

In August, Jonathan Oberlander (2008) published an article in the *New England Journal of Medicine* titled "The Partisan Divide—the Mc-Cain and Obama Plans for U.S. Health Care Reform." Oberlander also saw the coming election as perpetuating a partisan divide over health care. "There is broad agreement that the U.S. health care system requires reform. However, Democrats and Republicans remain sharply divided over how to reform, as evidenced by the health care plans offered by the parties' presidential candidates. The ambitious reform agendas of Senators John McCain (R-AZ) and Barack Obama (D-IL) would take the U.S. health care system in very different directions" (p. 781). Oberlander went on to describe the central policy changes each of the candidates' plans proposed, characterizing each as "sketches rather than finished portraits, with many important details yet to be revealed." He concluded his analysis by suggesting that "whoever wins the presidency can expect fierce opposition to any attempt at comprehensive reform" (p. 784).

By September 2008, each candidate had received the formal nomination of his party. Each made clear that reforming the national health care system would be one of his top priorities as president. It did not take long for the partisanship that Oberlander had predicted to appear. A group of three conservative commentators, including Gail Wilensky, a former Medicare administrator under the first President Bush and an adviser to the McCain campaign, sharply criticized Obama's emerging plan (Antos, Wilensky, and Kuttner 2008): "The health reform plan put forth by Sen. Barack Obama . . . greatly increases the federal regulation of private insurance but does not address the core economic incentives that drive health care spending. This omission along with the very substantial short-term savings claimed raise serious questions about its fiscal sustainability" (p. w462).

In October, a week before the election, the *JAMA* provided each candidate a forum to present their plans. John McCain (2008) described his in the following terms:

> The foundation of my health care plan is a belief that American families—not government bureaucrats or insurance companies—should choose the coverage that best meets their unique needs . . . [T]he road to real reform does not lead through Washington and an expensive, bureaucratic, government-controlled system.
>
> To make insurance affordable for all Americans, I will provide a refundable tax credit of $2500 for individuals and $5000 for families to use for health insurance. People who currently get their health insurance through their employer would see little change and would continue to keep their coverage or investigate other options that might better fit their needs.
>
> Opening the health insurance market to nationwide competition would give people many more choices of policies that aren't burdened by expensive state regulations that drive out competition and drive up prices.
>
> My record in Washington has been one of working consistently across party lines to get things done. Health care reform is an issue that cannot be accomplished without reaching across the aisle.

Barack Obama (2008) likewise outlined the main provisions of his plan:

> The Obama-Biden plan will guarantee that all Americans have quality health coverage and will save a typical American family up to $2500 every year on medical expenditures . . .
>
> Americans will also be able to choose from a range of private health insurance options through a new National Health Exchange, which will establish rules and standards for participating plans. The Exchange will also include a new public plan that will provide coverage similar to the kind members of Congress give themselves.
>
> In addition, the Obama-Biden plan will require coverage for all children and require that employers either make a meaningful contribution to coverage for their employees or contribute a percentage of payroll toward the cost of the national plan.

This is our moment to turn the page on the failed politics of yesterday's health care debates and finally bring together business, the medical community, and members of both parties around a comprehensive solution to our health care crisis.

Notably, although the plans proposed by each of the candidates differed fundamentally in their approaches to expanding access to health insurance for the American public, each candidate closed his proposal by promising collaboration. McCain committed to "working consistently across party lines to get things done" and "reaching across the aisle," while Obama committed to "bring together . . . members of both parties around a comprehensive solution to our health care crisis." Each candidate pledged to avoid the sharp political divide that had sunk the Clinton health reform plan and delayed the renewal of SCHIP.

President Obama's Approach to Health Care Reform

Shortly after Barack Obama was elected president, the *Lancet* again addressed his proposal for health care reform (2008b, p. 1707): "A palpable sense of optimism, 'opportunity, and unyielding hope' has emanated from the USA since President-elect Barack Obama's victory speech on the historic night of Nov 4 . . . Health, currently one of the most divisive of political issues, could become a symbolic uniting force for the new administration."

One week after the election, the *New York Times* reported that Senator Max Baucus, the Democratic chairman of the Finance Committee, would release his own vision of reform (Pear 2008): "Aides to Mr. Obama said they welcomed the Congressional efforts, had encouraged Congress to take the lead and still considered health care a top priority, despite the urgent need to address huge problems afflicting the economy." Facing the severe economic downturn of the Great Recession, President Obama relied on members of Congress to hammer out legislation that included the reforms he had outlined during his campaign.

In his plan, titled *Call to Action—Health Reform 2009*, Senator Baucus reported that he had been working with other senators for six months to develop a plan that had bipartisan support. "In preparing to act, I led the U.S. Senate Finance Committee in holding nine hearings on health care reform this year and hosted a day-long health summit in June 2008 to explore in greater depth the problems plaguing our health system. I have spent a good deal of time talking to colleagues on both sides of the aisle and to stakeholders in the health care industry to get their perspectives on the issues that matter" (Baucus 2008). Baucus described his plan as follows (p. iv):

> The Baucus plan would ensure that every individual can access affordable coverage by creating a nationwide insurance pool called the Health Insurance Exchange. Those who already have health coverage could keep what they have. But for those who need affordable, guaranteed coverage, the Exchange would be a marketplace where Americans could easily compare and purchase the plans of their choice . . . While the Exchange is being created, the Baucus plan would make health care coverage immediately available to Americans aged 55 to 64 through a Medicare buy-in.

In formulating this plan, Baucus had worked closely with his Senate Finance Committee colleagues from both political parties with the goal of winning bipartisan support.

In January, several days before President Obama's inauguration, two members of the House of Representatives published their own health reform proposal. Jim Cooper, a Democrat from Tennessee, and Michael Castle, a Republican from Delaware, titled their publication *Health Reform: A Bipartisan View* (2009). These congressmen introduced their proposal in a very positive light.

> This optimistic assessment of the prospects for health reform from senior Democratic and Republican congressmen spells out several reasons why reform can be achieved early in the first year of the Obama administration. Political and policy factors suggest that President-elect Barack Obama is in a much better position than his predecessors to achieve comprehensive health reform, including universal coverage . . . [A]fter decades of frustration and disappointment, policymakers should set aside

their differences and enable the United States to join the ranks of developed nations by making sure every American has health insurance. (p. w169)

The congressmen cited their backing of the Wyden-Bennett Healthy Americans Act, which had been introduced in the Senate during the previous session of Congress by Senators Ron Wyden, a Democrat from Oregon, and Bob Bennett, a Republican from Utah. The proposed legislation had eight Democratic cosponsors and nine Republican cosponsors, as well as wide bipartisan support in the House. In providing both caution and advice to their congressional colleagues, Cooper and Castle observed, "Another oft-voiced excuse for the prospective failure of reform is that partisan bickering will make reform impossible." They suggested that "from a practical standpoint alone, nothing will pass the Senate without the sixty votes needed to cut off a filibuster; at present, Democrats will occupy no more than fifty-nine seats" (p. w170).

By the time of his inauguration on January 20, 2009, President Obama had assembled a highly talented White House staff to assist him in securing congressional approval of his plan for health care reform. The staff included experienced professionals such as Peter Orszag in the Office of Management and Budget and Ira Magaziner as his chief health policy advisor. This was a key tactical decision. "There are other reasons to be hopeful about reform. One is that the incoming administration appears to have learned from the Clinton administration's misadventures in health care reform." Based on the advice he had received from his staff, it was the president's clear intention "to work closely with Congress in crafting reform legislation rather than imposing a top-down plan" (Oberlander 2009, p. 322).

SCHIP Renewal as a First Step for the Obama Administration

The repeated veto by President Bush of bipartisan legislation that would have renewed and revised the SCHIP program helped to set the stage during the run-up to the 2008 elections. Health care was a major issue for both Barack Obama and John McCain. With the election of President Obama and the increase in the Democratic majorities in both the House and the Senate, one of the first issues the new Congress took up was renewal of SCHIP.

Congress took action on SCHIP even before President Obama was inaugurated on January 20. On January 13, one week after the new Congress had convened, Representative Frank Pallone of New Jersey introduced the Children's Health Insurance Program Reauthorization Act of 2009 (CHIPRA) in the House of Representatives. The proposed legislation was essentially the same as the previous SCHIP reauthorization passed by Congress in 2007 but vetoed by President Bush. On January 14, the very next day, the House approved CHIPRA by a vote of 289-139, with 40 Republicans joining 249 Democrats in support.

The Senate Finance Committee had also taken up SCHIP reauthorization and passed the proposal on January 15 by a vote of 12-7. In so doing, the Finance Committee elected to include in the bill a change that had been made in the House version, approved the day before, that covered legal immigrant children and pregnant women under SCHIP. Previously, these immigrants had been required to wait five years after entry into the United States to qualify.

The decision to add this provision to the Senate version annoyed some senior Republican members of the Finance Committee. "The nearly five-hour markup turned contentious at points, with Republicans, including ranking member Charles E. Grassley of Iowa, charging that Democrats had shut them out of the process and betrayed compromises worked out in the 110th Congress. 'It makes me damned disgusted,' Grassley told the panel. 'We had all sorts of cooperation . . . Now it's kind of feeling like you're thrown overboard'" (*CQ Almanac* (2009a). Most of the Republicans on the committee opposed early coverage for legal immigrants.

The bill was then sent to the full Senate for discussion and a vote. Republicans unsuccessfully tried to amend the bill to cap eligibility for families at 300% of poverty. Senator Grassley again brought up the early eligibility for legal immigrant children. Despite his objection, however, the change was included in the final version of the bill. The

Senate passed the bill on January 29 by a vote of 66-32, with 9 Republicans joining 57 Democrats. Senator Grassley voted against, voicing his opinion that the bill did serious damage to the bipartisanship that had helped get it passed under President Bush.

On February 4, the House then took up the Senate version of the bill, similar in most ways to the House version passed earlier, voting 290-135 to approve. That same day, the CHIPRA bill was taken directly to the White House, where President Obama immediately signed it. The bill provided four additional years of funding. It also changed the name of the program from the State Children's Health Insurance Program to the simpler moniker of the Children's Health Insurance Program, or CHIP.

When President Obama signed the CHIPRA legislation, he "said that the bill was a 'critical first step' to covering uninsured children and towards providing healthcare insurance for all Americans" (Tanne 2009a, p. 372). In a commentary published in the *New England Journal of Medicine*, John Iglehart (2009, p. 857) cautioned about the implications of the Democrats' success in getting SCHIP renewed, "The rapidity with which Democrats managed to reauthorize SCHIP should not be taken as a sign that it will be easy to pass broader proposals for expanding coverage to other uninsured populations . . . Moving on to more ambitious reforms will be more difficult, given the rapidly increasing federal deficit, the competing claims for federal resources, and the determination of Republicans to forestall the growth of public insurance."

Oberlander and Lyons (2009, p. w407) echoed this caution: "Those looking for reasons to be hopeful about comprehensive reform's political prospects during the Obama administration can take comfort in elements of the reauthorization story . . . Yet the SCHIP fight also provides ample warning signs about the difficult road ahead. The SCHIP reauthorization debate once again revealed the ideological divide in U.S. health policy . . . [A]lthough SCHIP expansion drew bipartisan support, the scope of that support was limited."

Moving on to Comprehensive Reform

It was President Obama's strategy to rely on congressional leaders to turn his general proposals for health care reform into specific legislation. Principal among them were Senator Baucus, chair of the Finance Committee, and Ted Kennedy, chair of the Senate Health, Education, Labor, and Pensions Committee. Both senators had experienced the frustration and disappointment of the failed Clinton health reform efforts in 1994. As reported by Oberlander (2009, p. 323), "Both senators are determined to move quickly, fearing that delay could dissipate momentum, as it did in 1993."

On February 4, President Obama signed the Children's Health Insurance Program Reauthorization Act of 2009, extending funding for CHIP for four years and broadening its eligibility criteria. On February 14, he signed the American Recovery and Reinvestment Act, which provided more than $700 billion to stimulate recovery from the Great Recession of 2007–8.

With these major legislative actions behind him, President Obama shifted his focus to his proposals for health care reform. "Obama hosted a health-care forum at the White House on March 5. Among the invited 150 participants was a bipartisan group of senators and representatives, health-industry officials, providers, and consumer advocates" (Bristol 2009, p. 881). President Obama and his advisors cast their net widely to build as broad a foundation of support as possible. He had begun to get pushback from some Republican members of Congress. One central player in this opposition was Representative Paul Ryan from Wisconsin, who complained that Obama's plan was part of an effort to nationalize health care in the United States. Rather than calling for a nationalized system of care, Bristol characterized the plan in a different light: "Obama's proposals in the main are calling for reasonable sacrifices to a broad range of health-system participants. The strategy is so far blunting major opposition from many of the forces that doomed the Clinton reform plan in the 1990s" (p. 882). One of those forces was the repeated description of Clinton's reform proposals as calling for nationalized health care.

President Obama continued his efforts to reach out to a wide constituency beyond Congress. One group he reached out to in earnest was the American Medical Association. "Addressing a meeting of the American Medical Association's policy making House of Delegates in Chicago on 15 June, President Barack Obama has asked for the association's support for his healthcare reform initiative . . . An AMA spokeswoman said that the association was waiting to see what plans emerged from Congress" (Tanne 2009b, p. 1522). As we will see, the AMA subsequently came out in favor of one of the key pieces of legislation under discussion in the House of Representatives.

In Tanne's assessment, President Obama's efforts to cultivate the endorsement of organizations such as the AMA were indicative of his clear intent not to repeat the mistakes of the Clinton administration. "The Clintons had laboured largely in secret, producing a complex, micromanaged package that Congress snubbed. But Obama, the 'yes we can' man, let the legislators work up the legislation . . . The process is more open this time. More measured, flexible, respectful of Congress" (Woodward 2010, p. E113).

Tanne reported that "unlike the Clinton administration 16 years ago, which submitted a highly detailed programme that failed, President Obama has not spelt out a programme. He has left that to Congress. Several proposed bills are working their way through the legislative process. At least three approaches have been presented in the House of Representatives and the Senate. The plans will be argued over during the summer, and legislation will be proposed for a vote in the early autumn" (2009b, p. 1522).

In addition to approaching organizations such as the AMA, President Obama also reached out to the American public. On August 15, he described the central elements of his proposal in an Op-Ed in the *New York Times* (Obama 2009):

> Our nation is now engaged in a great debate about the future of health care in America . . . There are four main ways the reform we're proposing will provide more stability and security to every American.

First, if you don't have health insurance, you will have a choice of high quality, affordable coverage for yourself and your family—coverage that will stay with you whether you move, change your job or lose your job.

Second, reform will finally bring skyrocketing health care costs under control, which will mean real savings for families, businesses and our government.

Third, by making Medicare more efficient, we'll be able to ensure that more tax dollars go directly to caring for seniors instead of enriching insurance companies.

Lastly, reform will provide every American with some basic consumer protections that will finally hold insurance companies accountable . . .

This is not about putting the government in charge of your health insurance . . . In the end, this isn't about politics. This is about people's lives and livelihoods.

The House of Representatives Takes Up the Challenge

After having addressed the renewal of CHIP and the financial relief legislation, Congress began to work on the legislation that would put in place the type of health care reform President Obama had been pushing for. The Democratic leaders in the House released their first draft of this legislation on July 14. Three House committees—Energy and Commerce, Ways and Means, and Education and Labor—began holding hearings and discussions on the proposed legislation. Democratic representative John Dingell from Michigan sponsored the proposed legislation, along with eight cosponsors, all Democrats. H.R. 3200, titled America's Affordable Health Choices Act of 2009, included these major provisions:

- Establishing a national health insurance exchange to provide individuals and employers access to health insurance coverage choices. One of the options in the exchange would be a public health insurance option, structured in a manner similar to Medicare

- Requiring qualified health insurance plans to provide a series of essential benefits and to limit out-of-pocket expenses to $5,000 for an individual and $10,000 for a family
- Limiting variation in premiums to those based on age or geographic area
- Prohibiting exclusions from health insurance coverage based on preexisting conditions
- Providing for a premium credit and a cost-sharing credit for low-income individuals and families who obtain health insurance through the exchange
- Requiring all employers to offer health insurance coverage to employees or to make contributions to the exchange for any employees obtaining coverage there (small employers are exempt from this requirement)
- Imposing a tax on any individual without health insurance coverage
- Expanding Medicaid eligibility for all low-income individuals and families
- Making a series of changes to Medicare that would affect payment, coverage, and access
- Imposing a surtax on individual modified adjusted gross income exceeding $350,000
- Establishing the Center for Comparative Effectiveness Research to conduct and support health care services effectiveness research

The House Ways and Means Committee took up consideration of H.R. 3200. The resulting process turned out not to be bipartisan (*CQ Almanac* 2009b). Republicans on the committee proposed a series of 32 different amendments, all of which were defeated by the Democratic majority. The committee approved H.R. 3200 on July 17 by a vote of 23-18, with all of the committee's Republicans voting against the legislation, along with three Democrats.

The Education and Labor Committee considered H.R. 3200 during a session that lasted through the night of July 16-17. The committee added a series of amendments that increased the number of people eligible for coverage through the health insurance exchange. The committee blocked Republicans' attempts to remove key portions of the bill, including the public option and the tax for those without coverage. The committee approved the bill on a vote of 26-22. As was the case in the Ways and Means Committee, all of the committee's Republicans voted against the legislation, along with three Democratic members in a breach of bipartisanship.

The Energy and Commerce Committee also began consideration of H.R. 3200 on July 16. A group of Democrats objected to a number of aspects of the proposed legislation. These Democrats were members of the Blue Dog Coalition, a group of fiscally conservative Democratic representatives who caucused together, in particular to discuss fiscal impacts of proposals. To pass through the committee, its chair, Henry Waxman, negotiated a compromise with the Blue Dogs to lower the level of premium subsidies provided through the exchange and reduce coverage requirements for small businesses. Responding to the Blue Dogs, the committee also changed the way the public option plan would pay health care providers, relying on negotiated payment rates rather than rates set by Medicare. In a concession to liberal Democrats on the committee, the Blue Dogs agreed to amend the Medicare Prescription Drug Act to permit Medicare to negotiate drug prices directly with pharmaceutical manufacturers. The committee passed H.R. 3200 on July 31 by a vote of 31-28. Once again, all the committee's Republicans voted against the bill, along with five Democrats. The four Blue Dogs who had reached a compromise with Chairman Waxman voted in favor of the bill.

Shortly before each of the committees released its final version of H.R. 3200, an important event occurred outside of Congress. As reported on July 17 in *Physicians News Digest* (2009), "Today, the American Medical Association sent a letter to House leaders supporting H.R. 3200, 'America's Affordable Health Choices Act of 2009.'" The article quoted AMA president James Rohack: "This legislation includes a broad range of provisions that are key to effective, comprehensive health system reform . . . We support passage of H.R. 3200, and we look forward to additional constructive dialogue as the long process of passing a health reform bill continues."

Shortly after the AMA announcement, another news story cast a very negative light on H.R. 3200. On August 7, in a Facebook post, "Sarah Palin, the Republican who ran for vice president on the losing McCain ticket and recently resigned as governor of Alaska, claimed that the reform package would set up 'death panels' that would deny care to her son with Down's syndrome and her elderly parents" (Tanne (2009c). Palin was referring to a section of the bill that would authorize payment for doctors to counsel patients who requested advice on issues such as living wills, hospice care, and end-of-life planning. The complaint over "death panels" spread nationally, principally among those opposed to President Obama's health care reform efforts.

Each of the three committees had submitted its version of H.R. 3200 by the end of July. It then became the job of the House Democratic leadership, under Speaker Nancy Pelosi, to merge the three versions of the bill to bring to the floor of the House for discussion. The leadership preserved the changes the Energy and Commerce Committee had made as part of its agreement with the Blue Dogs. The leadership also included expansion of eligibility for Medicaid to those earning up to 133% of the FPL, up from 100%. The leadership bill also added a 2.5% tax on a range of medical devices to generate additional income for the premium subsidies through the exchange. The leadership maintained the public option to offer insurance coverage through the exchange.

In a controversial move, at the insistence of a number of moderate and conservative Democrats, Speaker Pelosi agreed to an amendment stipulating that no federal funds be used to provide abortion, with the usual exceptions for rape, incest, or danger to the mother's life. "In a deal that outraged House liberals, Pelosi agreed to a demand by Bart Stupak, D-Mich., to add tougher anti-abortion language. Stupak said that without his language, up to 40 Democrats might vote against the bill" (*CQ Almanac* 2009b). This change also had the backing of most Republicans. "Many abortion-rights backers unhappy over the outcome ultimately swallowed hard and voted for the amended bill."

The modified version of the bill was now labeled H.R. 3962. It came to a final vote by the full House on November 7 and was approved by a vote of 220-215. The work done by Speaker Pelosi to address the concerns of more moderate Democrats won her all but 39 Democratic members of the House. One Republican also voted in favor of the legislation.

The Senate Drafts Its Own Version of Health Care Reform

Two committees in the Senate took on the task of drafting legislation enacting the principles and goals outlined by President Obama: the Health, Education, Labor, and Pensions (HELP) Committee and the Finance Committee. As mentioned earlier, each of these committees had a leader who was firmly committed to passing health care reform legislation—Ted Kennedy of HELP and Max Baucus of Finance. When Senator Kennedy's developed malignant brain cancer, Christopher Dodd of Connecticut became the acting committee chair.

The HELP Committee began working on the legislation in June. It held a series of meetings, in which members proposed nearly 500 amendments. The committee accepted about 160 amendments that had been proposed by Republicans. On July 15, it approved its final version of the bill, S. 1679, by a strict party-line vote of 13-10. The bill included many of the same elements as H.R. 3962, including the government-run public option that would compete with private plans in the health insurance exchange. The Senate version proposed that the exchange be state based rather than national. As it was not within its assigned jurisdiction, the committee did not address changes to Medicare or Medicaid. That was the job of Finance.

Senator Baucus was the chair of the Finance Committee, and his colleague Charles Grassley from Iowa was the ranking member of the Republican minority. In sharp contrast to the partisan approach leaders of the House committees had taken, Senators Baucus and Grassley began working collaboratively early in the legislative process. A history of the health care reform process published by the Senate Finance Committee provides a detailed listing of its bipartisan meetings (2009).

As I described earlier in this chapter, approximately one week after Barack Obama was elected president, Senator Baucus issued a white paper titled his *Call to Action* for health care reform (2008). On April 21,

2009, Baucus and Grassley jointly led a Finance Committee roundtable, in which committee members met with health policy experts and industry representatives to discuss the options for health care reform. A week later, on April 29, Baucus and Grassley jointly released a list of policy options for consideration (Senate Finance Committee 2009).

Senators Baucus and Grassley held two additional roundtables, publishing an updated set of policy options following each. It seems clear that, while the Democrats and Republicans on the three House Committees that considered health reform legislation split sharply across party lines, the leaders of the Senate Finance Committee were making a sincere effort to maintain cross-party collaboration and respect.

In June, the bipartisan collaboration between Baucus and Grassley expanded to include six members of the Senate Finance Committee—three Democrats (Baucus, Kent Conrad of North Dakota, and Jeff Bingaman of New Mexico) and three Republicans (Grassley, Olympia Snowe of Maine, and Mike Enzi of Wyoming). Between June and September, this Gang of Six held a series of about 30 meetings, with the goal of developing draft legislation that would get at least some Republicans on board.

On September 22, a week after the final meeting of the Gang of Six, Baucus released his "chairman's mark" of the America's Healthy Future Act of 2009. The full committee then set to work on a final version that could muster committee approval.

On October 13, the full Finance Committee approved its bill, now labeled S. 1796, by a vote of 14-9. As described in the CQ *Almanac* reporting of these proceedings (2009b), "In the end, Snowe was the only Republican to vote for the committee bill, and she made it clear that she might not back the bill on the floor if it underwent changes. But the measure still reflected many of the group's compromises and was seen as the only version that had a chance on the Senate floor."

The Finance Committee's final bill differed in a number of important ways from the bills approved by the Senate HELP Committee and the three House committees. S. 1796 dropped the public option in the insurance exchange and replaced it with the option of consumer-owned, nonprofit health cooperatives offered on individual state exchanges. It also strengthened the employer mandate by requiring large and mid-sized employers either to provide affordable health insurance for all regular workers or to pay a fee for each employee who elected instead to obtain coverage through the state exchanges. The Congressional Budget Office (CBO) evaluated the potential long-term impacts of the proposal. Its report predicted that although the bill would cost nearly $900 billion over a period of 10 years, the increased revenues in the bill would result in a decrease in the federal deficit of $81 billion. The CBO also predicted that the bill would extend health insurance to 94% of Americans under the age of 65.

Harry Reid, the Senate majority leader, worked with the chairs of the HELP and Finance Committees to craft a final version of the bill to take to the floor. Unfortunately, the bipartisanship reflected in the negotiations of the Gang of Six had collapsed. As described by Wynne (2019), "Initial bipartisan negotiations led by Finance Committee Chairman Max Baucus had disintegrated, in part due to Tea Party–driven protests at Republican town-halls over the August recess." Up until the actual passage of the bill, Reid was unsure whether he could muster the 60 votes necessary to overcome a Republican filibuster. He worked with the two Democratic senators who had not committed their votes, Joe Lieberman of Connecticut and Ben Nelson of Nebraska. He had to reassure both senators that the final legislation would *not* include a public option, nor would it open Medicare enrollment to people aged 55–64, as many other Democrats had called for. Senator Nelson also insisted that, to secure his vote, the legislation needed to contain the same restrictions on abortion funding that Congressman Stupak had successfully added to the House version. In the end, Reid gained the votes of these two senators, assuring him of the 60 votes he needed.

The US Constitution requires all revenue bills must be initiated in the House and then passed on to the Senate for review and approval. Because the proposed health reform legislation involved substantial revenues, the Senate was prohibited from initiating the bill. To bypass this obstacle, Senator Reid elected to take H.R. 3590, a minor piece of legislation passed previously by the House, and to amend it so it contained instead the health reform bill the Senate had developed over these many months. The amended bill was now named the Patient Protection and Affordable Care Act.

Reid introduced H.R. 3590 for consideration in the Senate on November 19, hoping that he could still obtain at least partial bipartisan support for the bill. It took Reid two days to get the 60 votes necessary to bring the bill up for discussion on the Senate floor. Senate minority leader Mitch McConnell of Kentucky began a concerted effort to stall consideration of the bill. After repeated attempts to block these stalling tactics, Reid was able to muster 60 votes to invoke cloture as of 1 a.m. on December 21. Because of the necessity of two minor procedural votes, Senator McConnell was able to further delay the final vote, while cloture was invoked two additional times. The final vote for the Patient Protection and Affordable Care Act came on Christmas Eve, December 24. The bill was approved by a vote of 60-39. Unfortunately, the bipartisanship evident in the early stages of drafting the Affordable Care Act had evaporated.

Special Election in Massachusetts Changes the Path for the Affordable Care Act

The Senate version of the Affordable Care Act was passed without the vote of Senator Ted Kennedy of Massachusetts. Senator Kennedy died of brain cancer on August 25, 2009. Massachusetts governor Deval Patrick appointed Paul G. Kirk, a former chairman of the Democratic National Committee, to replace Kennedy in the Senate on a temporary basis until a special election to replace Kennedy could be held in January. Senator Kirk was one of the 60 votes Harry Reid needed to invoke cloture and gain final Senate passage of the Patient Protection and Affordable Care Act.

The special election in January was to change the political situation dramatically and contribute to the complex process through which President Obama managed to pass what is now commonly referred to as Affordable Care Act. Scott Brown, a Republican who had campaigned in opposition to it, was elected as a senator. With this change, the Democrats' Senate majority was reduced to 59 seats, one short of the number necessary to block a filibuster.

Recall that in November the House had passed H.R. 3962, its version of the health care reform law. H.R. 3962 differed in a number of ways from the law passed by the Senate. In the normal course of events, the House and Senate would have appointed a joint conference committee to negotiate a compromise bill for final discussion and approval by both the House and Senate.

With the Republicans now holding 41 seats in the Senate, they would have been able to block final Senate approval of the House/Senate compromise legislation through use of a filibuster. Democratic congressional leaders conferred and decided on an alternate means of passing the law. While the House version differed in a number of ways from the Senate version, its core components were largely the same as those in the Senate version. If the House were to pass the bill the Senate had approved without any amendments, the bill could then be sent to President Obama for his signature.

House Democratic leaders agreed to take this step on the assurance from Senate leaders that the Senate would pass a second bill that contained most aspects of the law that had been in the House version but not the Senate version. Congressional rules allowed a law to be passed with a simple majority of 51 votes in the Senate under the reconciliation process if it addresses only issues of financing. Reconciliation bills are not subject to a filibuster.

It took the House and Senate Democratic leaders more than two months following the election of Scott Brown in Massachusetts to gather the votes from their members to pursue this course. On March 21, by a vote of 219-212, the House passed the bill that had been approved by the Senate on December 24. On March 23, President Obama signed the Patient Protection and Affordable Care Act into law.

Thirty-four House Democrats had voted against the bill, along with all House Republicans, indicative of the disagreement that remained among House Democrats. The principal changes they had requested include the following:

- Increased support for health insurance premiums and limits on out-of-pocket costs for individuals and families under 400% of FPL
- Reduced tax liability for individuals who do not obtain health insurance coverage
- Increased penalties for large employers whose workers go to the health exchange for coverage
- Reduced costs for Medicare beneficiaries who hit the "donut hole" in pharmaceutical coverage under Medicare Part D
- Increased federal share of costs for coverage under the Medicaid expansion
- Increased Medicaid payment rates for primary care providers in 2013 and 2014

Each of these changes deals with issues of financing. To qualify for consideration under the reconciliation processes, the bill must address only financial issues. The Library of Congress (Health Care and Education Reconciliation Act 2009–2010) provides a more detailed description of the changes in this reconciliation act, labeled H.R. 4872.

On March 17, the House Budget Committee submitted a recommendation to the full House regarding proposed financial changes to the Affordable Care Act. On March 21, the report was considered by the House under rules that limited debate and prohibited amendments. At 11:36 p.m. on that same day, the House passed H.R. 4872, the Health Care and Education Reconciliation Act of 2010, by a vote of 220-211.

On March 23, the Senate took up consideration of H.R. 4872. Between March 23 and March 25, Republican senators proposed more than 30 amendments. Democrats either defeated or tabled discussion on each. Democrats were successful in making a few minor amendments to the bill, necessitating its return to the House for final consideration after passage in the Senate. Final Senate approval came on March 25 by a vote of 56-43.

The bill was forwarded to the House on the same day at 6:40 p.m. The full House then passed the bill at 9:02 p.m. that same day and forwarded it to the president. Obama signed the Health Care and Education Reconciliation Act of 2010 on March 30. The Affordable Care Act was then complete, with some portions of the law becoming effective immediately and the major portions of the law that created the health insurance exchanges and expanded Medicaid eligibility set to take effect in 2014.

Perhaps not unexpectedly, many Republicans reacted in anger over the way the Democrats had forced the original law through the Senate and then used the reconciliation process to amend it. On March 26, Senator John Cornyn, a Republican from Texas who served on the Senate Finance Committee, posted some very critical remarks on his office's website (2010): "The $3.4 trillion federal taxpayers spend on the Medicaid program is a target for waste, fraud, and abuse. Instead of fixing these problems, the President's new health care overhaul includes the largest expansion of the broken Medicaid program since its creation in 1965: it's only going to get worse from here." On March 21, Congressman Michael McCaul, a Republican from Texas, posted comparable criticisms on his website (2010): "In a purely partisan fashion, the Democrats have now passed the largest tax increase in history, a massive expansion of entitlements, and policies which will put the health care system at the whim of the Federal Government. One of the most distressing aspects of this legislation is the dishonesty which has been utilized for its passage."

Congressman McCaul's characterization of the Democrats' actions in passing the Affordable Care Act as "dishonesty" reflects the sharp divide between congressional Republicans and Democrats that resulted from its passage. As described by Weissert and Weissert in their book *Governing Health: The Politics of Health*, "When the health reform bill passed the Senate in 2010, using the reconciliation process to avoid a GOP filibuster, Republican Senators were so angry that they refused to participate in further legislative business, effectively shutting down the Senate" (2019, p. 107).

In first proposing the Affordable Care Act, President Obama made a sincere effort to craft a bipartisan plan to reform American health care. Leaders in the Senate worked consistently over a period of several months to involve both Democrats and Republicans in drafting the initial legislation. The Gang of Six, made up of three Democratic and three Republican senators worked tirelessly to craft a bipartisan approach to health care reform. In the end, these efforts to maintain bipartisanship failed. As described at the end of the previous chapter, President Bush's 2009 veto of the SCHIP renewal created a schism between the parties, "a division into mutually opposing parties of a body of persons that have previously acted in concert." By the time the Affordable Care Act was passed in 2010, that cross-party schism had only deepened. As we will see in the next chapter, that schism was to widen throughout the remainder of President Obama's term in office.

FOUR

Growing Congressional Opposition to the Affordable Care Act

AS DESCRIBED in the previous chapter, the Affordable Care Act was created through congressional approval of two separate pieces of legislation: the Patient Protection and Affordable Care Act, signed by President Obama on March 23, 2010, and the Health Care and Education Reconciliation Act of 2010, signed by President Obama on March 30.

Republican opposition to the ACA was immediate and widespread. On March 23, the same day President Obama signed the ACA, the attorney general of the State of Florida filed a lawsuit in federal court challenging its constitutionality. In rapid succession, 12 other states' attorneys general joined Florida as plaintiffs challenging the Affordable Care Act on the grounds that it exceeded Congress's authority within the commerce clause of Article I to regulate interstate commerce, and specifically that the individual health insurance mandate enforced by a tax penalty did not fall within Congress' authority to regulate interstate commerce. The suit also alleged that the individual mandate penalty did not fall within Congress's power to tax.

On January 31, 2011, the US District Court for the Northern District of Florida ruled in favor of the plaintiffs, agreeing that the ACA exceeded Congress's constitutional authority. The court also ruled that, because the individual mandate was unconstitutional, the entire ACA was unconstitutional because of the concept of "non-severability," that is, the court could not separate one part of the law from the entire law in determining its constitutionality.

The Obama administration appealed this ruling, and the 11th Circuit Court of Appeals concurred with the lower court that the ACA's individual mandate violated the Constitution. However, the appeals court found that the constitutional violation of the individual mandate did not make the rest of the ACA unconstitutional, in other words, the individual mandate was "severable" from the remainder of the law (*Florida v. U.S. Department of Health and Human Services* 2011).

As the lawsuit was making its way through the district court and the court of appeals, 13 additional states joined the lawsuit as plaintiffs along with the National Federation of Independent Business, a private organization "dedicated to being . . . the voice of small business" (n.d.). In the appeals process this lawsuit was merged with the suit filed by the states. The lawsuit reached the Supreme Court as *National Federation of Independent Business v. Sebelius* (*SCOTUSblog* 2012).

An additional complaint included in the lawsuit by the states proved to have substantial impact on the outcome. As discussed in chapter 2, Congress created Medicaid as part of the Social Security reforms passed in 1965. Under Medicaid, poor adults who were neither elderly (age 65 or greater) nor disabled could receive coverage only if they had children in their household younger than 18. Non-elderly, nondisabled, poor adults without children were not eligible. The ACA fundamentally changed this state of affairs. It required all states that were previously participating in Medicaid to expand eligibility for coverage to all adults who were poor or near-poor, with incomes less than 133% of the federal poverty line. (Because the method Medicaid uses to calculate income differs somewhat from the way income is calculated in determining the FPL, the federal government agreed to cover all people under 138% of FPL.)

Under previous coverage, the federal government reimbursed states for between 50% and 76% of the costs of caring for Medicaid beneficiaries, with higher reimbursement rates for states with lower per-capita incomes. Under the new coverage policy, which would take effect on January 1, 2014, the federal government would initially reimburse states for 100% of the cost of care provided to newly eligible adults, with the rate gradually decreasing to 90% by the year 2020. Following 2020, it would remain at 90%.

The ACA made this coverage expansion mandatory for all states. Those states that did not adopt this new eligibility for adults with incomes less than 138% of FPL would forfeit federal reimbursement for all coverage, including the elderly and disabled, under the original Medicaid law. In their lawsuit, the states contended that this new requirement to expand eligibility or lose all federal reimbursement was onerous to a degree that was prohibited by the Constitution.

The Supreme Court issued its ruling on June 28, 2012. "The Court agreed that the interstate commerce clause of Article 1, Section 8, did not apply to the decision to purchase health insurance, as individual decisions of this type are not part of interstate commerce. However, while the federal government may not force someone to acquire health insurance, it can levy an extra tax on those who elect not to obtain coverage. Even though ACA legislation identified the required payment as a 'penalty,' it was included under the federal government's authority under Article 1, Section 8, to 'lay and collect taxes'" (Barr 2016, p. 14). Congress may not force someone to acquire health insurance, although it can levy a tax on those who do not have insurance.

Regarding the challenge to the expansion of Medicaid under ACA, the court ruled that cutting off all Medicaid funding to any state that elected not to expand the program was a form of fiscal coercion that was not permitted under the Constitution. The Medicaid expansion could go forward under the law but would apply only to those states that elected to expand (Kaiser Family Foundation 2012).

The states that had filed the suit against the ACA had hoped to have the Supreme Court declare the entire law unconstitutional. By a narrow court majority, they were not successful in attaining this outcome. The principal outcome of their suit was to make Medicaid expansion optional for the states. As of 2020, 38 states and the District of Columbia had adopted the Medicaid expansion, while 12 states had not (Kaiser Family Foundation 2020).

Efforts in Congress to Weaken or Revoke the Affordable Care Act

While the lawsuits hoping to revoke the ACA were moving through the courts, the 2010 midterm election campaigns were taking shape. Many candidates focused their campaign on attacking the ACA. When the results were in, it was clear that the issue had flipped a number of Democratic congressional seats. In the Senate, the Democrats went from 59 to a smaller majority of 53. In the House, Republicans regained a majority with 242 seats as compared to 193 seats for the Democrats.

In 2017, the Congressional Research Service published a report titled *Legislative Actions in the 112th, 113th, and 114th Congresses to Repeal, Defund, or Delay the Affordable Care Act* (Redhead and Kinzer 2017a). In the introduction, the authors report that "Congress is deeply divided over implementation of the Affordable Care Act (ACA), the health reform law enacted in March 2010 during the 111th Congress. Since the ACA's enactment, lawmakers opposed to specific provisions in the ACA or the entire law have repeatedly debated its implementation and considered bills to repeal, defund, delay, or otherwise amend the law" (p. 1).

When the 112th Congress convened on January 3, 2011, it elected Representative Eric Cantor, a Republican from Virginia, as majority leader. Cantor immediately introduced H.R. 2, the Repealing the Job-Killing Health Care Law Act. As described by Redhead and Kinzer (2017a, p. 20), "H.R. 2 would have repealed the ACA in its entirety and restored the provisions of law amended or repealed by the ACA as if it had not been enacted." On January 19, the full House approved H.R. 2 by a vote of 245-189. When it reached the Senate, it was rejected by a vote of 47-51.

In April, Representative Fred Upton, a Republican from Michigan, introduced H.R. 1213, To Repeal ACA Funding for Health Insurance Exchanges. Shortly thereafter, Representative Michael Burgess, a Republican from Texas, introduced H.R. 1214, To Repeal ACA Funding for School-Based Health Center Construction, and Representative Joseph Pitts, a Republican from Pennsylvania, introduced H.R. 1217, To Repeal the Prevention and Public Health Fund. Each bill would have repealed essential components of the ACA. After rapid consideration, the House voted

- on April 13 to approve H.R. 1217 by a vote of 236-183,
- on May 3 to approve H.R. 1213 by a vote of 238-183, and
- on May 4 to approve H.R. 1214 by a vote of 235-191.

Each was rejected by the Senate, where the Democrats maintained a majority.

This process continued throughout 2011 and into 2012. When the Supreme Court issued its ruling at the end of June 2012 upholding the constitutionality of the ACA, Representative Cantor once again introduced a bill to repeal the ACA. His bill, H.R. 6079, the Repeal of Obamacare Act, would have invalidated the entire ACA. On July 11, the House approved the bill by a vote of 244-185. As with the previous bills, it was not approved by the Senate. H.R. 6079 was the 33rd attempt by congressional Republicans to repeal or substantially weaken the ACA, none of which became law.

On November 6, 2012, the nation reelected Barack Obama president by an Electoral College margin of 332-206, defeating his Republican opponent, Mitt Romney. In Congress, the Democrats increased their Senate majority slightly, from 53 seats to 55, including two Independent senators who caucused and usually voted with the Democrats. In the House, the Republicans lost several seats to Democrats, reducing their majority from 242 seats to 234, with Democrats holding 201 seats.

In the House, Republicans continued their efforts to repeal the ACA. Representative Michele Bachmann, a Republican from Minnesota, introduced H.R. 45, To Repeal the Patient Protection and Affordable Care Act. As with the bills from the previous Congress, this one was approved in the House by a margin of 229-195 only to face defeat in the Senate. The Republicans tried several more times over the summer of 2013 to repeal the ACA, each time failing in the Senate.

By the end of the summer, it was time for Congress to undertake its usual authorization of overall federal spending for fiscal year 2014, which was to begin on October 1. As a revenue measure, the Constitution requires that such legislation originate in the House. The House passed a resolution authorizing federal funding, with the exception that it revoked authorization for any funding of the ACA, scheduled to go into operation on January 1, 2014. The Senate considered the House funding resolution, passing it only after removing that provision.

When the resolution was returned to the House, the provision to revoke funding for the ACA was restored. Having previously voted to include funding for the ACA, the Senate elected to not even bring the repeat House bill up for discussion. The House and Senate were in a standoff over ACA funding, with authorization for federal funding to run out on September 30.

On October 1, lacking congressional authorization to fund its expenses, the federal government went into a shutdown. Without a funding authorization, the federal government was forced to furlough several hundred thousand employees without pay. Other essential employees were asked to stay at work without any salary. With most of the ACA covered by funding permanently authorized as part of the original legislation, the health insurance exchanges created by the ACA opened as scheduled.

The government shutdown was complicated by the fact that the Treasury Department was very close to the maximum debt permitted under law (the "debt ceiling"). Without a resolution to extend the debt ceiling, the government would have been unable to borrow the money necessary to cover its ongoing expenses.

As reported in the *New York Times* on October 16 (Weisman and Parker 2013), "Congressional Republicans conceded defeat on Wednesday in their bitter budget fight with President Obama over the new health care law as the House and Senate approved last-minute legislation ending a disruptive 16-day government shutdown and extending federal borrowing power to avert a financial default with potentially worldwide economic repercussions." It had taken pressure from Mitch McConnell, the Senate Republican minority leader, on House Speaker

John Boehner and his colleagues to back down on their efforts to block funding for the ACA. The Senate voted 81-18 to extend funding through January 15. The House then voted 285-144 to approve the Senate plan. President Obama signed the legislation shortly after midnight on Thursday, October 17. Only 87 House Republicans voted to approve the spending bill. They were joined by 198 Democrats in the final approval.

As I discussed at the end of the previous chapter, the Democrats' use of a combination of the original ACA legislation and the reconciliation act passed after the Democrats lost their 60-vote margin in the Senate angered many Republications. That anger led to a clear schism between the parties regarding the ACA. The schism was felt not only in Congress but among the states as well, and it led to repeated partisan battles. The lawsuits brought by a majority of the states led to the Supreme Court ruling in *National Federation of Independent Business v. Sebelius* that the ACA was constitutional, so long as each state had the option of expanding Medicaid coverage under the ACA.

The congressional bickering over ACA funding only added to the depth of the schism between the parties. By the time of the government shutdown in October 2013, the Republican House had voted a total of 46 times to repeal the ACA, either partially or completely. The October funding shutdown, at that time the second longest in history, only intensified the bitterness between the parties in Congress.

Efforts Outside of Congress to Weaken the ACA

With the Democrats still holding a majority in the Senate, the House was unable to take any action to weaken or delay implementation of the ACA. By 2013, Republicans in Congress as well as conservative organizations outside of Congress sought ways to block its implementation. One organization that took the lead in this effort was the Competitive Enterprise Institute (CEI). As described on its website, "CEI believes business leaders must play a larger role in challenging government intervention and special interest cronyism." With financing from the CEI, on May 2, 2013, Michael Carvin filed a lawsuit in the US District Court for the District of Columbia, *Halbig v. Burwell*. As Sarah Kliff reported (2015), "The Competitive Enterprise Institute, a Washington-based think tank, had financed the lawsuit and recruited a plaintiff (Jacqueline Halbig von Schleppenbach, a former Bush administration official turned consultant) for the case."

As described by the Federalist Society (n.d.), "In his 35 years at the Justice Department and in private practice, Mike Carvin is one of the leading appellate and trial lawyers challenging state and federal regulations on constitutional and statutory grounds . . . His major cases include the recent constitutional challenge to the Affordable Care Act." (The site also notes that "Mike was one of the lead lawyers, and argued before the Florida Supreme Court, on behalf of George W. Bush in the 2000 presidential election Florida recount controversy.")

The issue Carvin challenged in *Halbig v. Burwell* was wording in the ACA that he interpreted as preventing the federal government from financing premium support for families earning between 100% and 400% of FPL who obtain their coverage on Healthcare.gov, the federally operated health insurance exchange that offers coverage options for individuals and families in states that had elected not to establish their own insurance exchange.

The ACA authorizes each state to establish its own health insurance exchange, from which state residents without other affordable options can acquire health insurance coverage and, if eligible, access federal financial assistance in paying their insurance premiums. For example, California established Covered California (https://www.coveredca.com/) as its state exchange. States are not required to establish their own exchange, however. For those that elect not to do so, the ACA authorizes the federal government to provide coverage for state residents through the federal exchange, HealthCare.gov.

As described by Jost (2014, p. 890), "The ACA permits the purchase of health insurance with premium tax credits through virtual marketplaces called exchanges. Section 1311 of the ACA provides that states 'shall' establish exchanges, but since Congress cannot literally require states to do so, section 1321 provides that if a state 'elects' not to establish the 'required' exchange, the Department of Health and Human Services shall establish 'such' exchange for the state."

However, Carvin and his colleagues found an inconsistency in the wording of the ACA. "Buried in the ACA section authorizing premium tax credits are two subsections, addressing the calculation of credits and defining months for which credits are available, that say that tax credits are available for individuals enrolled in a plan 'through an exchange established by the state under 1311'" (Jost 2014, p. 890). The Internal Revenue Service (IRS) had concluded that those without a state exchange who obtain coverage through the federal HealthCare.gov exchange are still eligible for tax credits to reduce their premiums. Carvin challenged that interpretation, arguing that HealthCare.gov was not "an exchange established by the state" and was therefore ineligible for that premium support. He asked the court to issue an injunction prohibiting the federal government from paying premium subsidies on behalf of anyone signing up for coverage with the federal exchange. By 2015, 34 states had elected not to establish their own exchange, thus relying on the federal exchange to provide coverage for their state residents.

As described by Kliff (2015), "The newly filed lawsuit moved slowly. It irked Mike Carvin, the lawyer on the suit, enough that he sent the district court's chief justice, Royce Lamberth, a letter asking him to reassign the case to one his colleagues. So Carvin filed yet another lawsuit in Virginia, King v. Burwell, on September 16, 2013." Carvin intentionally filed *King v. Burwell* in Virginia rather than Washington, DC, to have two different appeals courts involved in case the lower court ruled against him. Once again, the CEI financed Carvin's lawsuit.

David King, the principal complainant in the suit, was a 63-year-old resident of Virginia. King was joined by three other Virginia residents as complainants: Douglas Hurst, Brenda Levy, and Rose Luck (*King v. Burwell* 2015). Each of the complainants was eligible under the ACA for the federal premium subsidy to purchase health insurance through an exchange. Because Virginia elected not to establish its own exchange, each would have had to go to HealthCare.gov to sign up for insurance eligible for that subsidy. None of the four wanted to do that, because without it, their incomes were low enough that they were exempt from the individual mandate under ACA. They argued that they preferred no insurance to insurance obtained from a federal exchange.

Interestingly, for *King v. Burwell*, several members of Congress filed amici curiae (friends of the court) briefs in support of the complainants, including Senators John Cornyn, Ted Cruz, Orrin Hatch, Mike Lee, Rob Portman, Marco Rubio, and Representative Darrell Issa. Senator John Cornyn also submitted an amicus curia brief in *Halbig v. Burwell*.

The federal judge hearing *Halbig v. Burwell* and the judge hearing *King v. Burwell* each ruled in favor of Sylvia Mathews Burwell, the defendant in both cases in her role as secretary of Health and Human Services. Both judges "held that the statute clearly authorizes federal exchanges to grant premium tax credits" (Jost 2014, p. 890). Attorney Michael Carvin rapidly filed an appeal in both of these decisions. His appeal of *Halbig v. Burwell* was heard on March 25, 2014, by the US Court of Appeals for the District of Columbia Circuit. His appeal of *King v. Burwell* was heard on May 14, 2014, by the US Court of Appeals for the Fourth Circuit.

On July 22, the Court of Appeals for the Fourth Circuit issued a unanimous verdict in *King v. Burwell* upholding the authority of the federal government to provide premium tax credits for those who enrolled in health insurance through HealthCare.gov. "The 4th Circuit observed that the ACA provision about the availability of Marketplace premium subsidies cannot be read in isolation from the rest of the statute. The 4th Circuit ruled that the ACA's language on this point is ambiguous and therefore the IRS has the authority to reasonably interpret the ACA" (Musumeci 2015).

On that same day, Court of Appeals for the District of Columbia issued its ruling in *Halbig v. Burwell*, determining by a vote of 2-1 that the language of the ACA is clear that in requiring that premium tax credits be provided only for individuals or families enrolled in state-based exchanges, it prohibited the use of premium tax credits for those enrolled in the federal exchange. "The DC Circuit found that the IRS rule contradicts the unambiguous wording of the ACA, and therefore the IRS overstepped its authority by allowing premium subsidies in states with a Federally-run Marketplace. The DC Circuit observed that when the language of a statute is clear, both the courts and administrative agencies must defer to the statute's plain meaning" (Musumeci 2015).

Jost (2014) also reported these contradictory decisions. Regarding the decision in *Halbig v. Burwell*, "Judge Thomas Griffith of the D.C. Circuit, writing for himself and Judge A. Raymond Randolph, decided that the phrase 'plainly distinguishes' state-operated from federally facilitated exchanges and allows only the former to issue premium tax credits" (p. 890). In the *King v. Burwell* decision, Jost writes, "Judge Roger Gregory, writing for the Fourth Circuit, similarly reviewed the wording of the premium-tax-credit provision and its context and history and concluded that neither side had clearly prevailed—although the government's arguments were better than the plaintiffs'. The courts must, he concluded, defer to the IRS interpretation of the statute and uphold the rule" (p. 891).

The plaintiffs in *King v. Burwell* appealed to the Supreme Court, asking it to overturn the decision of the Fourth Circuit. "The U.S. Supreme Court's surprise announcement on November 7 that it would hear King v. Burwell struck fear in the hearts of supporters of the Affordable Care Act (ACA). At stake is the legality of an Internal Revenue Service (IRS) rule extending tax credits to the 4.5 million people who bought their health plans in the 34 states that declined to establish their own health insurance exchanges under the ACA" (Bagley, Jones, and Jost 2015, p. 101). While the Supreme Court considered *King vs. Burwell*, the appellants in the *Halbig v. Burwell* case put their appeal on hold.

The Supreme Court heard arguments on March 24, 2015, and issued its decision on June 25, 2015. "For the second time in 3 years, U.S. Chief Justice John Roberts wrote a Supreme Court opinion that averted a near-death experience for the Affordable Care Act (ACA) . . . Writing for a six-member majority that also includes Justices Anthony Kennedy, Ruth Bader Ginsburg, Sonia Sotomayor, Stephen Breyer, and Elena Kagan, Roberts ruled that the ACA's tax subsidies for insurance premiums are available both in states with their own insurance exchanges and those relying on a federal exchange" (Hall 2015, pp. 497–98).

In the court's opinion, Roberts wrote, "When read in context, the phrase 'an Exchange established by the State under [42 U.S.C. §18031]' is properly viewed as ambiguous. The phrase may be limited in its reach to State Exchanges. But it could also refer to all Exchanges—both State and Federal—for purposes of the tax credits. If a State chooses not to follow the directive in Section 18031 to establish an Exchange, the Act tells the Secretary of Health and Human Services to establish 'such Exchange.' §18041. And by using the words 'such Exchange,' the Act indicates that State and Federal Exchanges should be the same" (*King v. Burwell* 2015, p. 3).

Hall (2015, p. 498) reported, "The Court ruled that Congress's actual intent can be honored because it's possible to read 'established by the State' to include federal exchanges operated as a fallback in states without their own exchange . . . [T]he Court stressed the need to consider the phrase in the context of the ACA's overall structure and purpose, rather than in isolation." In its closing remarks, the court made this position clear (*King v. Burwell* 2015, p. 21), "Congress passed the Affordable Care Act to improve health insurance markets, not to destroy them. If at all possible, we must interpret the Act in a way that is consistent with the former, and avoids the latter." In his commentary on this ruling, Hall (2015, p. 497) labeled the Supreme Court's decision as "ACA Armageddon averted."

The House of Representatives Files
Its Own Lawsuit against the ACA

In the months leading up to the launch of the ACA, the Obama administration made some changes to certain regulations in the law to facilitate its implementation. An important change of this type was the decision to delay enforcement of the employer mandate. As described by Stephen Redhead and Janet Kinzer, researchers for the Congressional Research Service, "On July 9, 2013, the IRS announced that it would not take any enforcement action against employers who fail to comply with the law's employer mandate until the beginning of 2015. This ACA provision, which took effect on January 1, 2014, requires employers with 50 or more full-time equivalent employees (FTEs) to offer their full-time workers health coverage that meets certain standards of affordability and minimum value." In addition to this initial delay, the Congressional Research Service reported, "The IRS subsequently announced that employers with at least 50 but fewer than 100 FTEs will have an additional year to comply with the employer mandate." The report characterizes these delays as "perhaps the most controversial administrative action taken by the Administration" because they were made without congressional approval (Redhead and Kinzer 2017, p. 2). However, the report goes on to explain why the Obama administration believed that these delays were necessary. "According to the Administration, these actions were taken after it was concluded that the ACA's employer mandate could not be enforced until the related requirement that employers report the coverage they offer to their employees had been fully implemented. The IRS indicated that it would work with stakeholders to simplify the reporting process consistent with effective implementation of the law" (p. 2).

A report by Ethridge (2013) quoted Mark Mazur, the assistant secretary for tax policy in the Obama Treasury Department, in explaining why the postponement was necessary: "The decision to delay the requirements was made after extensive conversations with stakeholders and a review of comments requesting a transition period . . . he said the delay will give the administration more time to find ways to simplify reporting requirements, and provides more time to adapt health coverage and reporting systems." Ethridge also described the reaction by congressional Republicans: "Several Republicans have questioned the administration's legal authority to delay enforcing certain provisions of the law . . . after the administration announced the postponement July 2."

Eilperin and Goldstein (2014) reported President Obama's decision to delay the employer mandate, as well as the public response to that decision in the *Washington Post.* "As word of the delays spread Monday, many across the ideological spectrum viewed them as an effort by the White House to defuse another health-care controversy before the fall midterm elections . . . Congressional Republicans seized on the announcement as the latest justification for scrapping the health-care law."

Congressional Republicans saw this alleged abuse of President Obama's authority under the ACA as an opportunity to mount a full-fledged attack against the ACA:

On July 30, 2014, the House voted 225-201 to approve a resolution (H.Res. 676) authorizing Speaker John Boehner, on behalf of the House, to sue the President or other executive branch officials for failing "to act in a manner consistent with [their] duties under the Constitution and laws of the United States with respect to implementation of the [ACA]." The Speaker indicated that any such lawsuit would specifically challenge the Administration's delay of the ACA employer mandate. "In 2013, the President changed the health care law without a vote of Congress, effectively creating his own law by literally waiving the employer mandate and the penalties for failing to comply with it," said Mr. Boehner. (Redhead and Kinzer 2017, p. 4)

H.R. 676 was introduced on July 22 and rapidly reviewed by the House Rules Committee before being passed by the full house on July 30. It "authorizes the Speaker of the House of Representatives to initiate or intervene in one or more civil actions, on behalf of the House . . . to seek any appropriate relief regarding the failure of the President . . . to act in a manner consistent with that official's duties under the U.S. Constitution and federal laws with respect to implementation of requirements of the Patient Protection and Affordable Care Act" (H.R. 676 2013–2014).

On November 21, 2014, the House of Representatives filed a lawsuit against President Obama and his administration—*U.S. House of Representatives v. Burwell.* The lawsuit claimed that the administration's delay of the employer mandates violated the US Constitution. The House added a second complaint to the suit, claiming that the administration was also violating the Constitution in paying cost-sharing subsidies to insurance companies under the ACA. "Unlike the premium tax credits, for which the ACA provided a permanent appropriation, the lawsuit argues that the law did not appropriate any funding for the cost-sharing subsidies" (Redhead and Kinzer 2017, p. 5).

The ACA exchanges offer four levels of health insurance coverage: bronze, silver, gold, and platinum, with each successive level covering a higher percentage of the cost of care along with carrying a higher monthly premium. Each plan has a deductible amount that the individual or family must pay out of pocket before the insurance would cover additional care. After the deductible is met, the insurance then pays a certain percentage of the cost of care, with the patient paying the balance as a copayment.

To make this insurance affordable to lower-income families, the federal government provides a tax credit to help pay the required monthly premium. Individuals and families making between 100% and 400% of FPL are eligible for this premium subsidy. To assist with the out-of-pocket costs incurred through the deductible and copayments, the ACA provides additional aid for individuals and families with incomes between 100% and 250% of FPL. The law also lowers the cap on total out-of-pocket spending for the year. To be eligible for these cost-sharing reductions, the individual or family would have to select a silver insurance plan. After the patient reaches the annual cost cap, their insurance company is responsible for paying health care providers for the patient's share of the cost of care. The federal government then reimburses the insurance company for these costs.

Republicans in Congress found an inconsistency in wording of the ACA legislation and the accompanying reconciliation act regarding tax credit premium subsidies and cost-sharing reductions. The ACA provides permanent funding for the Department of Health and Human Services (HHS) to pay the premium tax credits (PTCs) for all individuals and families between 100% and 400% of FPL. HHS does not have to request funding for the premium tax credits from Congress as part of the yearly budget allocation process. The Republicans discovered, however, that the wording of the legislation did not explicitly apply that same permanent finding to fund reimbursement of health insurance companies for the extra costs they must pay for those patients who have reached the out-of-pocket maximum for the year. The law is explicit that the insurance company must cover these costs for those patients who exceed the limit, but the law does not describe the mechanism through which HHS will acquire the funding to cover these costs.

Alissa Dolan, a legislative attorney working with the Congressional Research Service, has reported that, under U.S. *House of Representatives v. Burwell*, "the House's first claim alleged that the Treasury, at the direction of HHS, expended funds that were not appropriated to it by Congress, in violation of various constitutional and statutory provisions" (2016, p. 3). Dolan goes on to describe the particulars of this claim:

> The ACA established two kinds of subsidies—premium credits and cost-sharing subsidies. Section 1401 provides refundable tax credits to be available for certain individuals to reduce the cost of their health insurance premiums, referred to as a premium credit . . . Certain individuals and families receiving the credits are also eligible for coverage with lower cost-sharing (i.e., out-of-pocket costs such as deductibles and copays) than otherwise required under the applicable health plan. Under Section 1402, health plans must reduce the cost-sharing for these enrollees. The affected insurance plans are then to be reimbursed by the Treasury in the same amount, through the provision of cost-sharing subsidies."
>
> The Section 1401 premium credits are funded through a permanent appropriation, outside the annual appropriations process, for refunds due under the Internal Revenue Code . . . In its complaint, the House argued that unlike the Section 1401 premium credits, the Section 1402 cost-sharing subsidies are subject to the annual appropriation process. The House has maintained that Congress did not appropriate funds for the cost sharing subsidies in the Fiscal Year 2014 appropriations process . . . Therefore, the executive branch was not authorized to make the cost sharing subsidy payments that began in January 2014.

The House argued that, since the Obama administration had been making these cost-sharing reduction payments starting January 1, 2014 without congressional authorization, it had violated Article I, Section 9 of the Constitution, which states that "No Money shall be drawn from the Treasury, but in Consequence of Appropriations made by Law."

According to Dolan (2016, p. 4), "The House's second claim concerned implementation of the so-called employer mandate, a provision of the ACA that imposes a penalty on certain employers who fail to offer full-time employees health coverage that meets certain standards of affordability and minimum value." The ACA explicitly states that these employer penalties shall apply starting January 1, 2014. As described above, the Obama administration had decided in January 2013 to delay these penalties for a year to give employers more time to develop the mechanisms for reporting their compliance with these requirements. In February 2014 it further delayed the penalties for midsized employers. The House claimed that the failure to enforce these payment requirements starting in January 2014 was, in essence, a rewriting of the ACA legislation without congressional approval.

Although the Supreme Court had previously granted individual members of the House of Representatives legal standing to file a lawsuit when they have been harmed as individuals, "*Burwell* is the first suit to examine congressional institutional plaintiff standing based on an injury unrelated to information access" (Dolan 2016, p. 6). Dolan goes on, "In response to the House's November 2014 complaint alleging multiple constitutional and statutory violations arising from cost-sharing subsidy payments and the delay in enforcement of the employer mandate, HHS and Treasury (the agencies) filed a motion to dismiss. The motion argued, in part, that the House lacked standing to bring such a suit" (p. 11). The district court ruled that "the House had standing to sue on its appropriations cost-sharing subsidy claim. However, the House was only granted standing to sue on its count alleging certain constitutional violations, and not on counts alleging statutory violations" (p. 14).

According to the ruling, the House had legal standing to challenge the payment to insurance companies for the cost-sharing reductions. It did not have standing to challenge the delay of the employer mandate. Accordingly, the court dismissed this section of the House's lawsuit. The trial went forward, and, as Dolan reports, "the court issued its opinion on the merits in May 2016, in which the House prevailed on its cost sharing subsidy claim" (p. 20). The Obama administration appealed this decision to the District of Columbia Circuit Court in July 2016. As we shall see in the following chapters, the election results of November 2016 were to powerfully impact the outcome of the lawsuit as well as the financial stability of the health insurance market nationally.

One might say that the failure to include a permanent budget allocation for the CSRs in the original ACA legislation was simply a glitch of the legislative drafting process. The drafters of the law didn't intend to leave out the permanent appropriation for the CSRs. It just slipped by them without them being aware of the consequences.

This wasn't the only glitch subsequently discovered in the ACA. In 2014, the first year of coverage under the ACA, employers, employees, and health policy analysts discovered another such problem—the "family glitch."

Earlier in this chapter I discussed the employer mandate that is part of the ACA. Under the mandate, employers with more than 50 full-time employees are required to offer health insurance that is affordable to their workers. If the insurance they offer isn't affordable, workers can then go into the health insurance exchange and select a plan that qualifies them for premium tax credits, so long as the worker's income is between 100% and 400% of FPL. "Based on the way eligibility for premium tax credits is determined under current Internal Revenue Service (IRS) regulations, employer-sponsored insurance, for both the employee and his or her family members, is deemed affordable if the cost of self-only coverage—that is, a plan that covers only the individual worker—is less than 9.50 percent of household income" (Brooks 2014, p. 1). The problem is that "defining eligibility in this way ignores the cost of a family plan, which is frequently much more expensive than self-only coverage" (p. 2). So long as the health insurance for the individual worker costs them no more than 9.5% of their income, that worker is not eligible for premium tax credits through the health insurance exchange. What, though, about the worker's family members? The way the ACA legislation was written disqualifies the worker's family from a premium tax credit subsidy through the exchanges so long as the individual worker's share of the premium is no more than 9.5% of income. Lower-wage workers may not be able to afford the cost of adding family coverage through work, yet those family members who otherwise would qualify for the tax credit through the exchange are barred from doing so. Brooks estimated that between 2 million and 4 million family members were caught in this glitch.

It would have taken a simple measure for Congress to amend the wording of the ACA to redefine "affordable" coverage for workers to make family members eligible for premium tax credits through the exchange. But by the time this glitch was discovered, Republicans held the majority in the House of Representatives and refused to take this otherwise simple step.

In her analysis of the "family glitch," Brooks concludes, "Whether an oversight or a drafting error, experts at every point along the political spectrum agree that the current interpretation unfairly penalizes families. However, there is no consensus on fixing the problem . . . Unfortunately, the current political polarization in Washington calls into question the probability of such action, especially when it comes to the highly contentious health reform law." On June 5, 2014, Senator Al Franken, a Democrat from Minnesota, introduced S. 2434, the Family Coverage Act, to fix the glitch and give workers' families access to affordable health insurance through the exchanges while the worker got affordable individual coverage through work. Republicans in the Senate blocked consideration of the bill, and it never came up for a vote. From the experience with the Franken bill, Brooks concludes (2014, p. 3), "As is often the case, fixing the problem through the legislative process comes with a price tag, which would further fuel political rancor over the health reform law."

The Elections of November 2014 and the Change in Congress

The expansion of health insurance coverage through the exchanges and the expansion of Medicaid eligibility first took effect on January 1, 2014. As described in the previous section, 2014 was a year of intense acrimony between the Republican-dominated House of Representatives and both the Democratic Senate and the Obama administration. The House filed the *U.S. House of Representatives v. Burwell* lawsuit on November 21, 2014. Not quite three weeks earlier, the country had held its national elections on November 4, 2014.

In these midterms, Republicans increased their majority in the House of Representatives, from 233 seats over 199 for the Democrats to 247 seats over 188 Democratic seats. The Republicans also flipped the leadership in the Senate. Prior to the election, Democrats held 55 seats, including two Independents who caucused with the Democrats. After the elections, Republicans gained a majority of 54 seats, with Democrats holding 46. Both the House and the Senate were under firm Republican majorities. This situation had a powerful impact on Republican efforts to weaken or repeal the ACA.

On January 28, 2015, during the first month of activity in the new Congress, Representative Bradley Byrne, a Republican from Alabama, introduced H.R. 596, To Repeal the Patient Protection and Affordable Care Act and Health Care–Related Provisions in the Health Care and Education Reconciliation Act of 2010. Congressional Research Service analysts Redhead and Kinzer observe (2017, p. 15), "H.R. 596 would have repealed the ACA in its entirety and restored the provisions of law amended or repealed by the ACA as if it had not been enacted." After rapid review by House committees, the bill was passed by the full House on February 3 by a vote of 239-186 and forwarded to the Senate. The Senate received the bill on February 4 and placed it on its legislative calendar. However, since the bill was the type of legislation that was not eligible for reconciliation, it was subject to filibuster in the Senate. With the Democrats holding 46 seats, they blocked full consideration of the bill.

Given the Senate Democrats' refusal to consider H.R. 596, the Republican leadership in the House took a different tack. On October 16, 2015, Representative Tom Price, a Republican from Georgia, introduced H.R. 3762, the Restoring Americans' Healthcare Freedom Reconciliation Act of 2015. "The bill would have repealed the following ACA provisions: individual mandate; employer mandate; Cadillac tax; medical device tax; automatic enrollment requirement for large employers; and PPHF [Prevention and Public Health Fund]" (Redhead and Kinzer 2017, p. 14). It would have eliminated penalties for the employer mandate, thus eliminating these incentives to provide coverage to employees, as well as eliminating the individual mandate. It also would have repealed "the premium tax credits; cost-sharing reductions; and the HHS Secretary's authority to determine individuals' eligibility to participate in an exchange and receive the tax credits and cost-sharing reductions [as well as] the IRS's authority to disclose taxpayer return information to HHS for eligibility determinations" (p. 21). It also would have repealed funding for the Medicaid expansion, essentially eliminating it.

On October 23, barely a week after being introduced into the House, the bill was approved by a vote of 240-189. Each of these proposed changes to the ACA dealt with funding for its various programs. Accordingly, when Senate took up the bill, it was considered to be a reconciliation bill and was exempt from being delayed by a filibuster, needing only 51 votes to win Senate approval.

While the House had been working on developing H.R. 3762, the Senate Finance Committee and Health, Education, Labor and Pensions Committee had been developing their own reconciliation bill to repeal as much of ACA as they could. When they took up H.R. 3762 as passed by the House, these committees amended it with a series of their own provisions that went even further in repealing core aspects of ACA. The full Senate took up the bill on November 18. After about two weeks of discussion and debate, the Senate approved a series of amendments to the original H. 3762 and on December 3 approved the amended bill by a vote of 52-47.

On January 6, Representative Price, the original sponsor of H.R. 3762, made a motion to approve the bill as amended by the Senate. About three hours later that same day, the House approved the Senate version by a vote of 240-181. After years of trying, congressional Republicans finally succeeded in passing legislation to repeal the central aspects of the ACA. On January 7, the House forwarded the approved legislation on to President Obama. The next day, January 8, to no one's surprise, President Obama vetoed the legislation. The House took up his veto message and after about three weeks' discussion, voted to override. With a vote of 241 to 186, it fell substantially short of the two-thirds majority necessary to override a presidential veto.

On the website maintained by House Republicans, Price stated, "The president's health care law is doing real harm—increasing premiums and out-of-pocket costs, reducing access to care, levying more taxes and regulations on an already weakened economy, and injecting unnecessary government involvement into the lives of the American people. This damaging law needs to be repealed, so we can put in place positive, patient-centered solutions that would actually expand access to quality, affordable health care choices for all Americans" (n.d.).

On January 9, Gardiner Harris reported President Obama's veto in the *New York Times* (2016):

> Mr. Obama's veto—only the eighth of his presidency—was expected . . . But it shows that nearly six years after its enactment, the health law remains one of the most divisive political issues of the Obama presidency. For many Americans, the health law is seen as costly, cumbersome and a government infringement on freedoms, even as it has spread health coverage to millions and ensured popular benefits like ending lifetime coverage limits and the denial of insurance for pre-existing medical conditions. This week's House vote was the 62nd to fully or partly repeal the health law but only the first that sent legislation to the president's desk."

Harris then quoted Paul Ryan, the Republican Speaker of the House: "We have now shown that there is a clear path to repealing Obamacare without 60 votes in the Senate. So, next year, if we're sending this bill to a Republican president, it will get signed into law. Obamacare will be gone."

Following the veto, it was clear that the results of the November 2016 presidential elections would have substantial impact on the direction the Affordable Care Act would take.

FIVE

Efforts to Repeal the Affordable Care Act following the Elections of 2016

IT SEEMS clear that the failed efforts of Republicans in Congress in January 2016 to repeal the Affordable Care Act through the reconciliation process left an even wider schism between the two parties than existed following the passage of the Affordable Care Act in 2010. This schism affected policy analysts outside of government as well.

In March 2016, Gail Wilensky, formerly the Medicare administrator under President George H. W. Bush, along with two other conservative scholars argues in a commentary in *JAMA* titled "Replacing the Affordable Care Act and Other Suggested Reforms" (Antos, Capretta, and Wilensky 2016, p. 1324) that, "because so much attention has been paid to the repeal of the ACA by those who have opposed it, we believe it is important to focus on a serious proposal that could both replace this law and provide additional measures of reform, especially to the health care entitlement programs. We believe our reform agenda represents such a proposal." The authors then describe a series of steps to replace key aspects of the ACA, such as capping the tax exemption of employer-sponsored health insurance, splitting Medicaid into two separate programs and shifting to per-capita funding rather than open-ended cost reimbursement, and shifting Medicare to a market-based program in which beneficiaries would receive a fixed subsidy and select among competing plans.

This opposition to the ACA was also evident among many Republican voters in the time leading up to the November elections. In October, a compilation of 14 national opinion polls on the public's perception of the future direction of health policy in the United States (Blendon, Benson, and Casey 2016) revealed that overall, voters nationally were divided over the effect the ACA had had on the country, with 39 percent indicating that it had been positive and 44 percent that it had been negative. When the researchers then linked respondents' views to their party affiliation, they found that 80 percent of Democrats thought that the ACA had been working well while 88 percent of Republicans maintained the opposite perspective. From these results the authors concluded that, "overall in terms of understanding the implications of the 2016 election for the future of health policy, it is important to recognize that future changes in health policy are related more to the extent of political polarization between the parties on health care issues than to the importance of the issue itself in deciding the 2016 election" (p. e37[8]).

The 2016 elections were held on November 8. As reported by the Federal Elections Commission (2016), Hillary Clinton received 65,853,516 votes, comprising 48.18% of votes cast, while Donald Trump received 62,984,825 votes, or 46.09%. Under the Electoral College system, these votes translated into 304 electoral votes for Trump and 227 for Clinton. Despite coming up nearly 3 million votes short in the popular election, Donald Trump was elected the 45th president of the United States.

In the congressional elections, Republicans lost six seats in the House, maintaining a 241-194 majority. Republicans in the Senate lost two seats but maintained a 52-48 majority. With 52 seats, the only way for the Republicans to make significant changes to the ACA was through the reconciliation process.

On November 16, eight days after the election, Jonathan Oberlander concluded a commentary in the *New England Journal of Medicine* titled

"The End of Obamacare" (2016, p. 1), "The ACA has achieved much, including a large reduction in the uninsured population. Still, it lacks strong public support and an organized beneficiary lobby, has encountered significant problems in its implementation, and has been enveloped by an environment of hyperpartisanship."

On November 28, Gail Wilensky suggested in *JAMA* that, given the election results (2017a, p. 22), "repealing some or most of the funding for the ACA would be relatively easy to accomplish." To this end, she urged congressional Republicans "to pass a reconciliation bill similar or identical to the bill passed approximately a year ago." However, she also offered congressional Republicans two pieces of cautionary advice. If they were successful in revoking funding for the ACA, "ensuring that 20 million newly insured individuals retain coverage will be more challenging." She also cautioned that "Democrats would do everything within their legislative power to block any Republican policy objectives."

Enacting a bill similar to the Restoring Americans' Healthcare Freedom Reconciliation Act of 2015 that President Obama had vetoed in January 2016 would eliminate the Medicaid expansion, the individual mandate, and the employer mandate, as well as premium tax credits and cost-sharing reductions. In a report published by the Urban Institute, Blumberg, Buettgens, and Holahan (2016) estimated the potential impacts:

- The number of uninsured people would rise from 28.9 million to 58.7 million in 2019, an increase of 29.8 million people (103%).
- Working families would comprise 82% of people becoming uninsured.
- There would be 12.9 million fewer people with Medicaid or CHIP coverage in 2019.

Cindy Mann, the director of the Center for Medicaid and CHIP Services under the Obama administration during the rollout of the ACA, cited similar figures. To prevent such outcomes, she suggested that "a major question for Congress and President-elect Trump is whether they will proceed with a repeal bill without a 'replacement' bill in hand" (Mann 2016). Wilensky (2017b) took to the pages of the *Milbank Quarterly* to echo Mann's apprehensions. Concerned about the momentum that seemed to be gathering among congressional Republicans, she worried that "the forces for 'repeal and figure out next steps later' may be too great for serious, bipartisan legislation—even if it complicates the ultimate goal of 'repeal and replace.'"

In December 2016, the US Department of Health and Human Services issued a report on the impacts of three years of the ACA on health insurance coverage. More than 10 million people had acquired coverage through the exchanges, and an additional 15.7 million had enrolled in Medicaid. It also reported that 2.3 million young adults were now covered through the ACA provision that allowed them to remain on their parents' health insurance through their 26th birthday. As a result of these increases in coverage, the report indicated that "the uninsured rate has fallen to the lowest level on record." Repealing the ACA, as the 2015 Republican reconciliation would have done had it not been for President Obama's veto, would have largely reversed these advances. Were the Republicans in Congress willing to take this step and take responsibility for these consequences? This question was of substantial concern for many people nationally.

On January 6, in his last weeks in office, President Obama cautioned in an article in the *New England Journal of Medicine* titled "Repealing the ACA without a Replacement—the Risks to American Health Care" (2017). President Obama warned that "this approach of 'repeal first and replace later' is, simply put, irresponsible—and could slowly bleed the health care system that all of us depend on . . . Put simply, all our gains are at stake if Congress takes up repealing the health law without an alternative that covers more Americans, improves quality, and makes health care more affordable" (p. 298).

On January 17, three days before President Trump's inauguration, at the request of the Democratic leadership in the Senate, the Congressional Budget Office (2017a) issued a report titled *How Repealing Portions of the Affordable Care Act Would Affect Health Insurance Cover-*

age and Premiums. The purpose of the report was to estimate what the impacts would have been if H.R. 3762 had been signed rather than vetoed by President Obama. The report concluded:

> In brief, CBO and JCT [Joint Committee on Taxation] estimate that legislation would affect insurance coverage and premiums primarily in these ways:
> - The number of people who are uninsured would increase by 18 million in the first new plan year following enactment of the bill. Later, after the elimination of the ACA's expansion of Medicaid eligibility and of subsidies for insurance purchased through the ACA marketplaces, that number would increase to 27 million, and then to 32 million in 2026.
> - Premiums in the nongroup market (for individual policies purchased through the marketplaces or directly from insurers) would increase by 20 percent to 25 percent . . . in the first new plan year following enactment. The increase would reach about 50 percent in the year following the elimination of the Medicaid expansion and the marketplace subsidies, and premiums would about double by 2026.

President Trump was inaugurated on January 20, 2017. On that same day he issued his first executive order (number 13765), "Minimizing the Economic Burden of the Patient Protection and Affordable Care Act Pending Repeal" (Trump 2017). The first words in that order state, "By the authority vested in me as President by the Constitution and the laws of the United States of America, it is hereby ordered as follows: Section 1. It is the policy of my Administration to seek the prompt repeal of the Patient Protection and Affordable Care Act (Public Law 111-148), as amended." Jost and Lazarus reported (2017, p. 1201), "Within hours after taking the oath of office, President Donald Trump executed his first official act: an executive order redeeming his campaign pledge to, on 'day one,' begin repeal of the Affordable Care Act (ACA)." Jost and Lazarus underscore that President Trump was not able under the law to repeal any part of the ACA by executive order. He had to rely on Congress to take on that job.

The House of Representatives Approves the American Health Care Act

Discussions among congressional Republicans on how best to repeal the ACA began as soon as the new Congress convened on January 3. On January 3, Senator Michael Enzi, a Republican from Wyoming who was chair of the Senate Budget Committee, introduced S.Con.Res. 3 to authorize the use of the reconciliation process to repeal parts of the ACA. Over vocal opposition on the part of Senate Democrats, the full Senate approved the resolution on January 13 by a vote of 51-48, with all Democrats voting against and all Republicans voting for, with the exception of Republican senator Rand Paul, who objected to the resolution's failure to balance the federal budget. On January 13, the House approved a similar concurrent resolution by a vote of 227-198, with nine Republicans joining Democrats in opposition. Concurrent budget resolutions do not require the president's signature. Rather, they set the procedural rules for proposed legislation.

As reported in the *New York Times* by Pear and Kaplan (2017), "House Republicans unveiled on Monday [March 6] their long-awaited plan to repeal and replace the Affordable Care Act, scrapping the mandate for most Americans to have health insurance in favor of a new system of tax credits to induce people to buy insurance on the open market. The bill sets the stage for a bitter debate over the possible dismantling of the most significant health care law in a half-century." The bill introduced into the House was titled the American Health Care Act (AHCA). It was immediately referred to the Ways and Means Committee and to the Energy and Commerce Committee, where each committee began its own markup of the bill. As reported by Jost (2017), "The committees will begin markup of the bills on March 8, 2017 . . . If the bills are passed by the committees they will be combined by the House Budget Committee and sent to the House Rules Committee, and then to the full House for a vote." Both articles comment on the fact that the House committees were developing their proposed legislation without the results of a CBO report on its expected impacts.

The House Ways and Means Committee approved its version of the American Health Care Act on the morning of March 9. That afternoon, the Energy and Commerce Committee passed its version. The two committee reports were then referred to the House Budget Committee for final drafting. On March 20, the Budget Committee reported out its final version, labeled H.R.1628, American Health Care Act of 2017, and forwarded the legislation to the House floor for discussion.

On March 13, the Congressional Budget Office issued its estimates of the fiscal impact of the American Health Care Act (2017b, p. 1): "CBO and JCT estimate that enacting the American Health Care Act would reduce federal deficits by $337 billion over the coming decade and increase the number of people who are uninsured by 24 million in 2026 relative to current law." It also predicted that premiums for private health insurance would increase by 15%–20% (p. 3). The CBO further pointed out how the loss of health insurance would not be experienced equally across the insured population: "Although the agencies expect that the legislation would increase the number of uninsured broadly, the increase would be disproportionately larger among older people with lower income; in particular, people between 50 and 64 years old with income of less than 200 percent of the FPL would make up a larger share of the uninsured" (p. 21).

On March 9, the *New York Times* published an article titled "Health Groups Denounce G.O.P. Bill as Its Backers Scramble" (Goodnough, Pear, and Kaplan 2017). Three of the leading health care reporters for the *Times* wrote:

> Influential groups representing hospitals and nurses came out on Wednesday against a Republican bill to repeal and replace the Affordable Care Act, joining doctors and the retirees' lobby to warn that it would lead to a rise in the uninsured . . . The groups, including the American Hospital Association, the Association of American Medical Colleges, the Catholic Health Association of the United States and the Children's Hospital Association, said they could not support the bill as currently written. The hospitals and the American Nurses Association

joined the American Medical Association and AARP, which rejected the bill on Tuesday.

Republican leaders in Congress were coming under increasing pressure to find a way to reduce the adverse impact of the ACA repeal legislation. On March 24, Erica Werner and Alan Fram (2017) reported for NBC News in Chicago that, "in a humiliating failure, President Donald Trump and GOP leaders pulled their bill to repeal 'Obamacare' off the House floor Friday when it became clear it would fail badly . . . Republicans had never built a constituency for the legislation, and in the end the nearly uniform opposition from hospitals, doctors, nurses, the AARP, consumer groups and others weighed heavily with many members."

After much discussion and negotiation among House Republicans, resulting in a series of amendments to the bill, on May 3 the House Rules Committee voted to return H.R. 1628, the American Health Care Act of 2017, to the full House for a final vote. On May 4, the House passed the bill 217-213, with 20 Republicans joining all 193 Democrats in opposition. It was then up to the Senate to take up the bill and try to find a path to final approval.

In May 2017, the Henry J. Kaiser Family Foundation, a nonpartisan, nonprofit health policy organization, produced a report detailing the specific actions taken under the American Health Care Act (2017):

- Repeal ACA mandates (2016), standards for health plan actuarial values (2020), and premium and cost sharing subsidies (2020)
- In 2020, replace ACA income-based tax credits with flat tax credits adjusted for age; phase out eligibility for new tax credits at income levels between $75,000 and $115,000
- Retain private market rules, including requirement to guarantee issue coverage, prohibition on preexisting condition exclusions, requirement to extend dependent coverage to age 26
- Retain health insurance marketplaces, annual open enrollment periods, and special enrollment periods
- Convert federal Medicaid funding to a per capita allotment and limit growth in federal Medicaid spending beginning in 2020,

using 2016 as a base year; states that had elected not to expand Medicaid could receive block grant funding to cover poor adults and children

- Add state option to require work as a condition of eligibility for nondisabled, non-elderly, nonpregnant Medicaid adults
- Prohibit federal Medicaid funding for Planned Parenthood clinics
- Prohibit abortion coverage requirements

On May 24, the CBO issued an updated report on the predicted impacts of the final version of the American Health Care Act that was approved by the House on May 4 (2017c). The updated report predicted that enacting the bill would reduce federal deficits by $119 billion over a period of 10 years and increase the number of uninsured by 23 million by 2026. It also indicated that health insurance premiums for single adults would increase by about 20% in 2018. Compared to the March 13 report, the final version of H.R. 1628 would have a somewhat smaller decrease in the federal deficit without substantially changing the number of people who would become uninsured or the increase in premiums for those who purchased health insurance.

The Senate Takes Up the Effort to Repeal the ACA

On May 4, the same day that the House passed the American Health Care Act, Bob Bryan (2017) reported that "Republican senators signaled they plan to almost completely gut the American Health Care Act and rewrite their own version of the bill after the AHCA passed the House on Thursday, a sign the fight over repealing and replacing Obamacare is far from over." Bryan reported that Senator Chuck Grassley, Republican chairman of the Finance Committee said that, rather than adopting the House's bill, the Senate would draft its own health reform bill.

On May 9, the *New York Times* reported that Senate majority leader Mitch McConnell of Kentucky had appointed "a 13-man working group on health care, including staunch conservatives and ardent foes of the

Affordable Care Act—but no women" (Pear 2017). Pear goes on to describe its makeup: "The Senate Republican working group on health care includes the party's top leaders, as well as three committee chairmen and two of the most conservative senators, Ted Cruz of Texas and Mike Lee of Utah." Senator McConnell included himself as a member of the working group, but he elected not to include either Senators Susan Collins of Maine or Lisa Murkowski of Alaska, both women having expressed a more moderate perspective on health care reform.

On June 1, Professor John McDonough of the Harvard School of Public Health commented in the *New England Journal of Medicine* on the process the Senate was adopting in crafting legislation to repeal the ACA (2017, p. 2501): "Like their House counterparts, Senate Republican leaders are working hard to devise a bill negotiated only among the 52 GOP members, involving none of the chamber's 48 Democratic caucus members . . . Leaders intend to bypass standing committees in passing their plan."

H.R. 1628, the American Health Care Act of 2017 as passed by the House was introduced into the Senate on June 7. It was held in abeyance as the working group appointed by the Republican Senate leadership wrote a substitute version of the bill. It was clear that a number of Senators had serious objections to many aspects of the House bill. Yaver (2017) reported that, "despite the lack of consensus within the party, Senator Mitch McConnell, the majority leader, on Wednesday began the process of fast-tracking the bill under Rule 14, which enables the Senate to bypass the committee process and instead move the bill on to the Senate calendar for a vote as soon as it is ready."

Very little information was made public about the changes the Senate would make to the House bill. The working group did its work behind closed doors. On June 13, the editorial board of the *New York Times* wrote in "The Senate Hides Its Trumpcare Bill Behind Closed Doors" (2017a), "A coterie of Republicans is planning to have the Senate vote before July 4 on a bill that could take health insurance away from up to 23 million people and make changes to the coverage of millions of others. And they are coming up with the legislation behind closed doors without holding hearings, without consulting lawmakers who disagree with them and without engaging in any meaningful public debate." The writers go on to make the point that "Mr. McConnell's strategy belies the disingenuous Republican complaint that Democrats jammed the A.C.A., or Obamacare, into law in 2010 without sufficient analysis or discussion." The editorial then cites the fact that the process of crafting the Affordable Care Act under President Obama lasted more than a year, during which time, "the House and Senate came up with several competing bills, held dozens of hearings, accepted Republican amendments and spent countless hours soliciting feedback from public interests groups and the health care industry."

The Republican leadership released a draft of its revised bill on June 22. The next day, the editorial board of the *Times* published a second editorial in response (2017b). It underscored the extent to which the Senate bill would seriously weaken Medicaid by shifting it to a per-capita reimbursement to the states that would eventually be limited in its growth to the overall rate of inflation in the economy. It would also substantially reduce the subsidies available through the exchanges for low- and middle-income individuals and families. The writers concluded by arguing that "Mr. McConnell seems determined to steamroll this travesty through the Senate before July 4, despite complaints by conservatives and moderates."

On June 22 Gail Wilensky commented in the *New England Journal of Medicine* regarding the slow pace of efforts to repeal the ACA (Wilensky 2017c, p. 2407): "My expectations about the ease and speed of passing an Affordable Care Act (ACA) replacement bill during President Donald Trump's first 100 days in office have not exactly come to fruition." She provided her perspective on the American Health Care Act as passed by the House, then provided some political advice to Republicans in the Senate:

> Unfortunately, the legislation passed by the House and being developed in the Senate suffers from the same problem that plagued the ACA: single-party support. Major social legislation that is written and supported by only one political party is unlikely to be accepted by the other party or to become a stable part of the legislative landscape. It is truly

astounding that having railed against the Democrats for having pushed the ACA through Congress on a single-party vote, Republicans are doing exactly the same now that they've taken over control of the government. And yet presumably, they expect the country's reaction and acceptance to be different. (p. 2408)

On June 23, the day after Wilensky's article was published, Antos and Capretta (2017a) reported in a blog post that, "yesterday, Senate Republican leaders released a discussion draft of their version of healthcare legislation, the Better Care Reconciliation Act (BCRA). Senate Majority Leader Mitch McConnell plans to put this legislation to a vote next week with the expectation of passing it." The version of the bill Senator McConnell's working group had developed was renamed the Better Care Reconciliation Act, to distinguish it from the House's bill.

On June 26, the Congressional Budget Office issued a report of the fiscal impact of substituting the Senate version of the legislation in place of the House version (2017d):

CBO and JCT estimate that enacting this legislation would reduce the cumulative federal deficit over the 2017–2026 period by $321 billion. That amount is $202 billion more than the estimated net savings for the version of H.R. 1628 that was passed by the House of Representatives. The Senate bill would increase the number of people who are uninsured by 22 million in 2026 relative to the number under current law, slightly fewer than the increase in the number of uninsured estimated for the House-passed legislation. By 2026, an estimated 49 million people would be uninsured, compared with 28 million who would lack insurance that year under current law.

The Kaiser Family Foundation (2017) summarized the key provisions of the Better Care Reconciliation Act:

- Repeal ACA mandates and cost-sharing subsidies
- Modify ACA premium tax credits starting in 2020
- Create a new association health plan option for small employers and self-employed individuals
- Retain health insurance marketplaces

- Convert federal Medicaid funding to a per-capita allotment and limit growth in federal Medicaid spending beginning in 2020
- Add a state option to require work as a condition of eligibility for non-elderly Medicaid adults who are not disabled or pregnant
- Repeal most ACA revenue provisions

By the middle of July, there still was no Senate version of the bill ready to introduce into the full Senate for debate. It wasn't until July 25 that Majority Leader McConnell introduced a motion to proceed to allow the Senate to consider the original House bill. When the final roll call vote was taken, the tally was 50 Senators voting in favor of discussing the House bill and 50 Senators voting against. This necessitated Vice President Mike Pence to cast the tie-breaking vote (Cong. Rec. 2017).

Following the motion to proceed, Senator McConnell proposed an amendment to H.R. 1628 to replace the House version of the bill with the Better Care Reconciliation Act drafted by his working group. It soon became clear to McConnell that he did not have sufficient support among Republicans to pass his amended bill. This became even more evident when Senator Cruz proposed an amendment to permit insurers to offer plans that don't cover essential health benefits or offer community rating, under which each person enrolling in the plan is charged the same premium based on age, two key components of the ACA. On July 25, when McConnell tried to get his bill passed, he failed by a vote of 43 in favor and 57 against. Those voting against the bill included nine Republicans.

Having earlier become aware of the growing resistance among moderate Republican senators to a repeal of the key aspects of the ACA, McConnell also prepared backup legislation that would modify the ACA without revoking major components. Labeled the Health Care Freedom Act, this draft legislation was humorously referred to as "skinny repeal." On July 26 McConnell introduced the act as a proposed amendment. Its key components included the following (Kaiser Family Foundation 2017):

- Repeal ACA individual mandates and suspend the employer mandate until January 1, 2025
- Retain private market rules, including requirement to guarantee issue coverage to any eligible applicant regardless of disease risk, set premiums based on modified community rating, prohibit preexisting condition exclusions, require coverage of essential health benefits, require dependent coverage be extended to age 26
- Retain health insurance marketplaces with annual open enrollment periods
- Modify certain provisions regarding ACA 1332 state innovation waivers to expedite the approval process and to permit waivers to be in effect for longer periods
- Retain the Medicaid expansion
- Prohibit federal Medicaid funding for Planned Parenthood clinics for one year
- Suspend imposition of the medical device tax for three years

The proposed law would have maintained the premium subsidies and cost-sharing subsidies. However, it would have simplified the granting Section 1332 state innovation waivers and would have authorized the granting of state waivers that would end or reduce federal subsidy payments to individuals and employers in the state. It would also have authorized $2 billion to help states draft and implement waiver proposals.

On July 27, the Congressional Budget Office (2017e) issued a brief summary of the impacts of the Health Care Freedom Act. The act was expected to increase the number of uninsured adults by 16 million by 2018 and reduce the federal deficit by approximately $17 billion by 2021.

Discussion of the Health Care Freedom Act on the Senate floor began on July 27. Democratic efforts to refer the bill to committees for further analysis were defeated. It then came up for a final vote on July 28, in what is perhaps one of the most graphically recognized Senate actions in recent memory. As the roll call vote proceeded, Republican senators Susan Collins of Maine and Lisa Murkowski of Alaska joined all 48 Democrats in voting against the motion, with 49 of the Republicans voting in favor. This left one senator to cast the deciding vote (American Health Care Act of 2017).

If the vote had been split at 50-50, Vice President Pence would once again have added his vote in favor of the motion to approve the bill. Senator John McCain of Arizona cast the deciding vote. Just a week before, McCain had been given a diagnosis of brain cancer. Having recently undergone surgery, he had nonetheless returned to Washington a few days earlier to cast this vote. As reported by Austin Ramzy in the *New York Times* (2017), "Mr. McCain left his intentions secret until the end, then cast his vote in a dramatic fashion, walking to the middle of the floor, holding his arm out and then giving a thumbs-down."

Three days earlier, McCain had given a speech on the floor of the Senate, chiding many of his Republican colleagues. As reported by Cowan and Oliphant (2017), "McCain took to the floor and urged his fellow Republicans to stand up to Trump, who has frequently chided the Republican-led Congress for failing to advance his agenda . . . Most of his remarks on Tuesday, however, were directed at his fellow senators. He blasted the process through which Senate Republicans crafted their healthcare legislation, shutting out Democrats and writing the bill out of public view. McCain has repeatedly said that Democrats did little better in 2010, when Obamacare was passed, and added, 'We shouldn't do the same with ours.'"

The Country Responds to the Republican Failure to Repeal the Affordable Care Act

Shortly after the failure of the Republican efforts to repeal the ACA, Jacob Pramuk (2017) reported a statement issued by the three Republican Senators whose votes defeated those efforts. "Sens. Susan Collins, R-Maine, Lisa Murkowski, R-Alaska, and John McCain, R-Ariz., said they still wanted to revamp the American health-care system to reduce costs and stabilize markets in pockets of the country. But they urged Senate leaders to take up an approach with both parties, rather than the Republican-only effort that characterized the various pushes to repeal or replace parts of the Affordable Care Act in recent weeks."

The American public as well as the national press were following the efforts by President Trump and by Republicans in Congress to repeal the Affordable Care Act. The failure of the Senate to pass any of the proposed options had a profound impact on the public's perception of the legislative process. Oberlander described the public response (2017a, p. 1001): "For 7 years, Republicans vowed to repeal and replace the Affordable Care Act (ACA) . . . Yet less than 7 months into the Trump administration, the GOP's crusade to dismantle Obamacare has, at least for now, collapsed." Oberlander described how, as Republicans battled among themselves, the public actually became increasingly aware of many of the benefits of the ACA that they might end up losing if key elements of the ACA were revoked. "Ironically, the GOP managed to increase support for the ACA, whose favorability improved markedly during the repeal-and-replace debate" (p. 1003). Oberlander concluded his analysis by providing some constructive advice to congressional Republicans: "Abandoning that commitment to repeal Obamacare, and instead working with Democrats on incremental measures to improve the law, will not be easy . . . But could it mark a turning point?" (p. 1003).

On August 30, governors from the states of Ohio, Colorado, Nevada, Pennsylvania, Alaska, Virginia, Louisiana, and Montana jointly submitted a letter addressed to Paul Ryan, Speaker of the House; Nancy Pelosi, House minority leader; Mitch McConnell, Senate majority leader; and Charles Schumer, Senate minority leader (Kasich et al. 2017). Three of the governors were Republicans and five were Democrats. The letter described the problems each state was facing in sustaining its health insurance system: "The current state of our individual market is unsustainable and we can all agree this is a problem that needs to be fixed. Governors have already made restoring stability and affordability in this market a priority, and we look forward to partnering with you in this effort."

Each of the states represented by these governors had elected to expand Medicaid as of 2018. None wanted its newly eligible Medicaid recipients to lose coverage. The governors offered three central recommendations to congressional leaders: "We recommend (1) immediate federal action to stabilize markets, (2) responsible reforms that preserve recent coverage gains and control costs, and (3) an active federal/state partnership that is based on innovation and a shared commitment to improve overall health system performance." The governors also offered specific recommendations on steps such as permanently funding cost-sharing reductions, maintaining the individual mandate, and fixing the "family glitch."

In September, Long et al. published new data on the success of the ACA in making health insurance more available nationally (2017, p. 1656): "Adults in all parts of the country, of all ages, and across all income groups have benefited from a large and sustained increase in the percentage of the US population that has health insurance. The gains have been particularly striking among low- and moderate-income Americans living in states that expanded Medicaid." The percentage of non-elderly adults who were uninsured had dropped from 17.6% at the end of 2013 (just before the ACA took effect) to 10.2% in the first quarter of 2017. The sharpest drop in the uninsured was in families with incomes at or below 138% of FPL—due largely to the expansion of Medicaid. Of those who remained uninsured, 60.4% lived in states that had elected not to expand Medicaid. As the authors concluded, "Scaling back the coverage options under the ACA would have serious health and financial consequences for some of the most vulnerable Americans, including older adults and adults with preexisting health conditions. Though the politics of health reform are challenging, there are opportunities to create a more equitable and efficient health care system by recognizing the ACA's achievements while addressing its problems" (p. 1661).

Despite the clear benefits of the ACA to millions of Americans and the repeated call for bipartisan cooperation to strengthen the health care system, Republicans in the Senate were not yet done trying to repeal substantial portions of the ACA. On September 13, Republican senators Lindsey Graham of South Carolina and Bill Cassidy of Louisiana submitted a proposed amendment to the American Health Care Act. Republican senators Dean Heller of Nevada and Ron Johnson of Minnesota joined as cosponsors. The proposed amendment became known as the Graham-Cassidy-Heller-Johnson (GCHJ) amendment.

According to the Kaiser Family Foundation (2017), GCHJ would have taken several major steps to roll back central provisions of the ACA. These included repealing the ACA individual and employer mandates and the funding of premium and cost-sharing subsidies; establishing a new state block grant program to provide $1.176 trillion over seven years to encourage state-designed health care reform programs; repealing the Medicaid expansion and converting Medicaid to per-capita funding; giving states the option to require work as a condition of Medicaid eligibility for non-elderly adults; and prohibiting federal Medicaid funding for Planned Parenthood clinics for one year.

Antos and Capretta (2017b) analyzed GCHJ, which they referred to as Graham-Cassidy: "The Graham-Cassidy plan is built on the premise that the federal government should remove itself from many of the difficult policy decisions concerning how health insurance is subsidized and regulated. Those decisions would be left to the states." The authors underscore that shifting federal assistance for acquiring insurance through the exchanges and for the Medicaid expansion to a new state block grant funding mechanism would result in a substantial redistribution of funding from higher-income states that had expanded Medicaid to lower-income states that had elected not to.

Under the Senate rules, any reconciliation bill had to be passed by September 30, the end of the fiscal year. With GCHJ first introduced on September 13, that gave Majority Leader McConnell very little time to allot to discussion and analysis of the bill. The Senate Finance Committee would get one day to review the proposed legislation. It would have to do so without an analysis by the Congressional Budget Office, as the time did not allow for that.

McConnell had announced that the Senate would vote on GCHJ in the week prior to September 30. However, several key senators publicly announced their opposition to the bill, including Rand Paul, John McCain, Lisa Murkowski, and Susan Collins. After considering the opposition he faced within his own party, on September 26, McConnell announced that the Senate would not vote on GCHJ. As reported on CNN (Fox et al. 2017), "The Senate will not vote on the Graham-Cassidy bill to repeal Obamacare, Republican leaders announced Tuesday, dealing a devastating blow to President Donald Trump and GOP lawmakers who tried to make a last-ditch attempt to deliver on the party's years-long campaign promise . . . Tuesday marked a clear end to the latest campaign to try to jam through a partisan bill to gut the Affordable Care Act."

Lessons Learned from the Failure of Efforts to Repeal the ACA

In April 2017, when it looked as though the House might fail in its attempt to pass the American Health Care Act, Jonathan Oberlander (2017b) attempted in the *New England Journal of Medicine* to put this potential failure in the broader historical context of efforts at national health care reform:

> Failure is a familiar outcome in U.S. health policy. Presidents have long struggled to translate their promises and aspirations into legislative victory. Harry Truman's national health insurance program never came close to becoming law. Richard Nixon's universal coverage plan did not pass. Congress rejected Jimmy Carter's hospital cost-containment bill. Bill Clinton's campaign to enact universal insurance ended in political disaster. Yet even judged against this dismal history, Republicans' March 2017 efforts to repeal and replace the Affordable Care Act (ACA) were an epic failure. (p. 1497)

Oberlander offered an explanation for this historical string of failures: "Hyperpartisanship has dented the ACA's political fortunes, complicated its implementation, and created an increasingly dysfunctional and conflict-ridden federal government" (p. 1497). From the day that President Obama succeeded in passing the Affordable Care Act, and subsequently the accompanying Health Care and Education Reconciliation Act, the Republicans in Congress drew a hard line between opposition to the ACA and bipartisan collaboration to improve problems with the ACA that appeared following its enactment. Over three subsequent Congresses and more than 300 efforts in the House to repeal the ACA, the opposites sides of that line became more and more widely separated.

After the election of President Trump and the bicameral Republican congressional majorities, Republican leaders made it clear they had no intention even to speak with their Democratic colleagues about the ACA repeal process. As the political schism over the fate of the ACA widened, those standing on either side had an increasingly hard time seeing those on the other side and reaching out to communicate with them.

In his analysis of the apparent failure in the House to repeal the ACA, Oberlander (2017b) made a prediction of what steps might come next: "If Republicans cannot pass repeal legislation, the Trump administration has other options to undermine Obamacare, including weakening enforcement of penalties for not obtaining insurance and eliminating federal payments to insurers that are required to provide cost-sharing subsidies to lower-income Americans for deductibles and copayments. Such actions could explode the individual insurance marketplaces." As we discover in the next chapter, Oberlander proved to be prescient.

| SIX |

Attempts by Congress and the Trump Administration to Disrupt ACA Financing

IN CHAPTER 4, we considered *U.S. House of Representatives v. Burwell*, the lawsuit the House of Representatives had filed against President Obama to stop funding payments to insurance companies to reimburse them for the cost-sharing reductions (CSR) that were required under the Affordable Care Act (ACA). To understand the full impact of the lawsuit and its outcomes, I will first describe the types of financial assistance individuals and families are eligible for under the ACA when they purchase their health insurance from an exchange, either a state exchange or Healthcare.Gov.

Those who purchase such a policy and who have incomes between 100% and 400% of the federal poverty line are eligible for a federally financed premium tax credit to help pay part of the monthly premium for the insurance. Based on the individual's or the family's income on the most recent year's federal tax return, the amount the family or individual will pay each year is capped at a certain percentage of their income. (The health insurance exchange links to the Internal Revenue Service database to determine this amount.) The maximum percentage of income to be paid out-of-pocket for health insurance premiums during 2019 is shown in table 6.1.

Table 6.1 Maximum Annual Health Insurance Premium Based on Income, 2019

Income as a percentage of FPL	Maximum annual premium as percentage of income
100%–133%	2.08%
133%–150%	3.11%–4.15%
150%–200%	4.15%–6.54%
200%–250%	6.54%–8.36%
250%–300%	8.36%–9.86%
300%–400%	9.86%
<100% or >400%	Ineligible for premium cap

Source: Kaiser Family Foundation 2018.

It should be noted that in 2019 the Trump administration announced that it would be changing the formula used to calculate the maximum out-of-pocket costs for monthly insurance premiums and for 2020, "the increased percentage would result in higher premiums for at least 7.3 million exchange consumers by cutting their premium tax credits" (Keith 2019a).

If an individual or family is eligible, the federal government will pay directly to the insurer the difference between the actual cost of the premium and the maximum premium based on the insured's income. The ACA specifies that the premium cost is calculated based on the second-lowest-cost silver plan available to the insured in the exchange marketplace. (Recall that market exchanges under the ACA offer four levels of coverage: bronze, silver, gold, or platinum.)

In its explanation of how these premium caps work, the Kaiser Family Foundation (2018, p. 4) provides the following example, using data for 2019:

- Pat is 30 years old and estimates her 2019 income will be 250% of poverty (about $30,350 per year).
- Suppose the second-lowest-cost silver plan available to Pat in the marketplace is $500 per month.
- Under the ACA, with an income of $30,350 per year, Pat has a cap of 8.36% of her income for that plan.
- This means that Pat would have to pay no more than $211 per month (8.36% of $30,350, divided by 12 months) to enroll in the second-lowest-cost silver plan.

- The tax credit available to Pat would therefore be $289 per month ($500 premium minus $211 cap).
- Pat can then apply this $289 per month discount toward the purchase of any bronze, silver, gold, or platinum marketplace plan available.

The federal funding for payments to health insurance companies for the premium amounts above the limits for eligible individuals and families was established as a permanent authorization under the ACA. Accordingly, no congressional action is necessary to authorize the administration to make these payments each year. As I discussed in chapter 4, however, individuals and families are eligible for another type of spending subsidy under the ACA: CSRs. The CSRs apply to additional out-of-pocket costs individuals or families face for expenses such as the annual deductible under their plan, coinsurance or copayments, and pharmaceuticals. These CSRs are available only to individuals and families with annual income between 100% and 250% of FPL. The out-of-pocket maximum for these costs, not including the health insurance premiums, is shown in table 6.2.

As with the premium tax credits described in table 6.1, individuals and families with incomes less than 100% of the FPL are ineligible for the cost limitation. When the ACA was first passed in Congress, all citizens and eligible permanent residents with incomes less than the FPL were covered by Medicaid, with no monthly premium or cost sharing. Accordingly, this group was left out of eligibility either for PTCs or CSRs. It was only after the Supreme Court made Medicaid expansion optional that poor individuals in states electing not to expand Medic-

Table 6.2 Maximum Annual Limitation on Cost Sharing, 2019

	Out-of-pocket maximum	
Income as a percentage of FPL	Individual	Family
<100%	$7,900	$15,800
100%–200%	$2,600	$5,200
200%–250%	$6,300	$12,600
>250%	$7,900	$15,800

Source: Kaiser Family Foundation 2018.

aid wound up ineligible not only for Medicaid but also for the PTCs and CSRs.

As described in chapter 4, those writing the actual text of the ACA left out some key wording. Whereas PTCs are covered by a permanent budget allocation, the legislation did not explicitly state that the CSRs would also be covered by a permanent allocation. When the Republican House of Representatives learned of the CSR glitch, it authorized the leadership to file a lawsuit against the Obama administration to stop these unauthorized payments. Accordingly, on November 21, 2014, the House filed the *U.S. House of Representatives v. Burwell* lawsuit, asking the court to prohibit the payment for CSRs.

The Obama administration claimed that the House lacks legal standing to file a lawsuit against the administration. On September 9, 2015, the federal judge issued a ruling "that the House had the right to sue the Obama administration over billions of dollars in health care spending, a decision that poses a new legal threat to the health care law and gave congressional Republicans a victory in their claims of executive overreach by the White House" (Hulse 2015).

The court then conducted a trial on the merits of the case, issuing its ruling on May 12, 2016. Robert Pear declared in the *New York Times* (2016), "Victory for House Republicans in federal court last week could mean significantly higher health insurance premiums for millions of people if the decision is upheld on appeal, the Obama administration said Monday . . . The ruling by Judge Rosemary M. Collyer of the United States District Court for the District of Columbia would block the administration from reimbursing insurers for discounts provided to millions of low-income people under the Affordable Care Act." On July 16, 2016, the Obama administration appealed the ruling. Accordingly, the judge stayed her injunction against making these payments until the federal appeals court decided the case.

As one might expect, the elections of November 2016 had a substantial impact on the case and the issues it was deciding. Donald Trump was inaugurated on January 20, 2017. On that same day, President Trump issued Executive Order 13675, Minimizing the Economic Burden of the Patient Protection and Affordable Care Act Pending Repeal (Trump 2017):

> Section 1. It is the policy of my Administration to seek the prompt repeal of the Patient Protection and Affordable Care Act (Public Law 111-148), as amended (the "Act").
>
> Sec. 2. To the maximum extent permitted by law, the Secretary of Health and Human Services (Secretary) and the heads of all other executive departments and agencies (agencies) with authorities and responsibilities under the Act shall exercise all authority and discretion available to them to waive, defer, grant exemptions from, or delay the implementation of any provision or requirement of the Act that would impose a fiscal burden on any State or a cost, fee, tax, penalty, or regulatory burden.

In November, President Trump announced that he intended to appoint Alex Azar, at that time President of the pharmaceutical manufacturer Eli Lilly and Company, to be his secretary of Health and Human Services, replacing Sylvia Burwell. Accordingly, Secretary Azar became the defendant in the suit by the House of Representatives, and the suit was referred to as *U.S. House of Representatives v. Azar*.

In light of the election of President Trump, the Republican leaders of the House decided to hit the pause button on their suit, which was originally filed against the Obama administration. As reported by Jost (2016a), "On December 5, 2016, the Circuit Court of Appeals for the District of Columbia acceded to the request of the House of Representatives and stayed further proceedings in House v. Burwell pending further motions by the parties, due by February 21, 2017 . . . This appellate court's order means that this lawsuit and its consequences are effectively no longer in the hands of the Obama administration and are now the full responsibility of the Trump administration and of Congress."

The two parties to the suit—the House of Representatives and the Trump administration—submitted further requests to stay the decision by the Court of Appeals, and the suit sat dormant for several months. Then, on August 1, 2017, 17 states and the District of Columbia entered motions to intervene in the suit. "The states had moved to intervene, claiming that they had an interest in the action and that the Trump administration was not adequately defending their interest . . . [T]he states had demonstrated that they had standing to intervene because they 'would suffer concrete injury if the court were to grant the relief the plaintiffs seek'" (Jost 2017a).

In December, the parties to the suit entered into a settlement. Again as reported by Jost (2017b), "The Trump Administration, House of Representatives, and attorneys general from seventeen states and the District of Columbia reached a settlement . . . The settlement would dismiss the appeal of the lower court's injunction blocking the cost-sharing reduction (CSR) payments, dissolve that injunction, and leave each of the parties to assert in future cases the positions they had taken in this litigation." This outcome left the Trump administration free to decide whether to terminate reimbursement to insurance companies for the CSRs they grant to eligible enrollees, since Congress had not authorized these payments.

The Impact of the Loss of Cost-Sharing Reductions on Health Insurance Premiums

It is important to underscore that, while the glitch in the ACA legislation did not grant permanent authorization for federal reimbursement of insurance companies for CSRs, the legislation still required insurers to grant CSRs to those enrollees who met two requirements: their income was between 100% and 250% of the FPL, and they enrolled in a silver plan. As shown in table 6.2, these enrollees had a maximum out-of-pocket payment for each year. Once they reached this level, they were no longer responsible for any out-of-pocket costs for any covered service for the remainder of that calendar year. The insurer was still obligated to reimburse the health care professional or organization providing these services their full cost as specified under the contract with the providers. Because the insurers had expected to receive federal reimbursement for these costs, those insurers had to find another way to make up for these lost costs.

The simplest way to recoup these costs was to raise the premiums for the silver-tier plans. In light of the uncertainty insurance companies faced in 2017, while the lawsuit was proceeding, most insurance companies made the decision to do precisely that for the 2018 calendar year, what has come to be known as "silver loading."

As early as 2016, before President Trump was elected, health policy analysts were speculating on what the impacts might be of ending reimbursement funding for CSRs. Gabel and colleagues (2016) issued a report on the potential impacts of the loss of those reimbursements: "Without the cost-sharing reductions (CSRs) made available by the Affordable Care Act, health plans sold in the marketplaces may be unaffordable for many low-income people." The authors pointed out that in 2016, 7 million people who were enrolled in health insurance through the exchanges were eligible for CSRs.

The Kaiser Family Foundation (2017) reported that "among 12.2 million people who selected a 2017 ACA marketplace plan, about 58 percent, or 7.1 million, are receiving cost-sharing reductions. An earlier Foundation analysis of 2017 plans found the subsidies lower combined medical and prescription drug deductibles by as much as $3,354 and reduce annual out-of-pocket maximums by up to $5,587." Taking these figures into account, "the average premium for a benchmark silver plan in Affordable Care Act (ACA) marketplaces would need to increase by an estimated 19 percent for insurers to compensate for lost funding if they don't receive federal payment for ACA cost-sharing subsidies."

Levitt, Cox, and Claxton (2017) emphasized that, as a result of the loss of federal reimbursement for CSRs, "insurers would only increase silver premiums . . . since those are the only plans where cost-sharing reductions are available." They also pointed out that "the premium increases would be higher in states that have not expanded Medicaid (and lower in states that have), since there are a large number of marketplace enrollees in those states with incomes 100–138% of poverty who qualify for the largest cost-sharing reductions." The authors estimated that, while silver plan premiums would increase by an average of 19% across all states, they would increase by 15% in states that had expanded Medicaid and 21% in states that had not.

Levitt, Cox, and Claxton (2017) made another key point: "While the federal government would save money by not making CSR payments, it would face increased costs for tax credits that subsidize premiums for marketplace enrollees with incomes 100–400% of the poverty level." Let us imagine a family that lives in a state that did not expand Medicaid and earns 125% of FPL. Since they are not eligible for Medicaid coverage, they must turn to the Healthcare.gov exchange to obtain their coverage. However, monthly premiums for silver-level insurance are going up by an estimated 21%. How can they afford these new premiums?

Recall from table 6.1 that a family that earns between 100% and 133% of FPL has their annual health insurance premiums capped at 2.08% of household income. Assuming their income did not go up, their maximum premium also did not go up. Yet the premium for coverage went up 21%. Who will pay that extra 21%?

The federal government will pay the full cost of the premium increase through the PTC for which the family is eligible. The irony of the decision by the Republican House of Representatives not to fund the reimbursement to insurance companies for the CSRs is that the federal treasury will instead have to pay the full cost of the increase in silver-tier premiums for all families with incomes between 100% and 400% of poverty, whether or not they are eligible for the CSRs. For each of these families, the annual premium is capped at the percentage of household income shown in table 6.1. Any family enrolling in a silver tier plan will face the substantially increased overall premium, but their share of the premium will remain the same. The federal government will pay the full cost of the increase. Levitt, Cox, and Claxton (2017) estimated that by not paying insurance companies directly for the CSRs, the federal government would save $10 billion in 2018; however, the government would have to spend an additional $12.3 billion for increased PTCs, for a net expenditure increase of $2.3 billion.

In August 2017, the federal Congressional Budget Office issued a report on "the effects of terminating payments for cost-sharing reductions" (2017). The CBO predicted as a result of the decision not to reimburse insurance companies for the lost revenue from the CSRs, "insurers in some states would withdraw from or not enter the non-group market because of substantial uncertainty about the effects of the policy on average health care costs for people purchasing plans" (p. 1). Furthermore, the report concurred with the previous study: "Because they would still be required to bear the costs of CSRs even without payments from the government, participating insurers would raise premiums of 'silver' plans to cover the costs" (p. 1). The CBO estimated that, for people with income between 100% and 200% of FPL, the reduction in CSR payments to insurance companies would be approximately equal to the increase in PTCs for this group, leading to no net change in federal expenditure. "However, increases in premium tax credits for those with income between 200 percent and 400 percent of the FPL would substantially exceed the small reductions in CSR payments for this group." Based on these factors, the CBO predicted that the overall effects of failure to pay the CSRs would include (p. 2):

- Gross premiums for silver plans offered through the marketplaces would be 20% higher in 2018 and 25% higher by 2020—boosting the amount of premium tax credits according to the statutory formula.
- Most people would pay net premiums (after accounting for premium tax credits) for nongroup insurance throughout the next decade that were similar to or less than what they would pay otherwise.
- Federal deficits would increase by $6 billion in 2018, $21 billion in 2020, and $26 billion in 2026.

In response to the CBO report, a *New York Times* headline trumpeted, "Trump Threat to Obamacare Would Send Premiums and Deficit Skyward." Robert Pear and Thomas Kaplan (2017) opened the article by declaring, "Premiums for the most popular health insurance plans would shoot up 20 percent next year, and federal budget deficits would increase by $194 billion in the coming decade, if President Trump carried out his threat to end certain subsidies paid to insurance companies under the Affordable Care Act, the Congressional Budget Office said Tuesday." The authors then quoted Representative Nancy Pelosi, the Democratic minority leader in the House who had originally requested the CBO report: "If he follows through with his threats, President Trump will be single-handedly responsible for raising premiums across America by 25 percent, exploding the deficit by nearly $200 billion."

The authors acknowledged the uncertainty of Trump's decision in light of these predictions by the CBO. "The Trump administration has been providing funds for cost-sharing subsidies month-to-month, with no commitment to pay for the remainder of this year, much less for 2018."

The answer to this uncertainty came on October 12, as reported by Margot Sanger-Katz (2017): "All year, President Trump had threatened to release a metaphorical bomb into the Obamacare markets—canceling a certain type of payment to health insurers. Everyone was convinced it would destroy the marketplace. Late last Thursday, he carried out his threat, later saying that 'the gravy train ended the day I knocked out the insurance companies' money.'"

Sanger-Katz (2017) made another point that few people were aware of at the time. Recall that, to receive CSRs, income-eligible families must enroll in a silver-tier plan. However, families making between 250% and 400% of FPL would not be eligible for CSRs, but they would still be eligible for the increased PTCs that came as a consequence of the insurance companies' loss of CSR reimbursement.

> For many Obamacare consumers, there's also a silver lining in these pricier silver plans. There are other kinds of plans being sold on the marketplace: high-deductible plans called bronze and low-deductible plans called gold and platinum. Consumers can use their subsidy to buy any color plan they like. And, with the price of silver plans rising faster than the other categories, most consumers with subsidies will now be able to buy a lower-deductible health plan for the same price as the silver plans that are currently most popular on the exchanges. (They can also choose to buy high-deductible bronze plans for very low prices, or in some cases get them free.)

Whereas the PTCs for which an individual or family is eligible are based on the premiums for the second-lowest-price silver plan offered on the exchange, referred to as the "benchmark plan," they can use these PTCs to purchase a plan at any of the four tiers: bronze, silver, gold, or platinum. To recoup the lost revenue from the failure of the Trump administration to pay for the CSRs, insurers were raising premiums substantially for the silver-level plans; however, premiums for the bronze, gold, and platinum plans were not affected. Accordingly, after applying the PTC calculated from the silver plan, an individual or family might find that the gold plan costs little more, or even no more, than the silver. The gold plan brings with it lower deductibles and copayments. This process of using increased PTCs for higher-priced silver plans to purchase plans at other levels is an important consequence of silver loading.

Rasmussen, Rice, and Kominski (2019) studied the population who obtained their coverage for 2018 through California's state exchange, Covered California. In response to the impacts of silver loading, they found that 7% of those who reenrolled in 2018 elected to change the metal tier of their coverage. Among those who changed tiers, 37% switched to a gold plan, leading the authors to conclude that "the implementation of silver loading discussed above provides evidence of a 'gold rush' among re-enrollees" (p. 1906).

Largely in response to the confusion caused by the failure of the federal government to fund CSR reimbursements, Qiu (2017) reported, "Senator Lamar Alexander, Republican of Tennessee, and Senator Patty Murray, Democrat of Washington, announced on Tuesday they had reached a compromise bill to continue the subsidies funding for two years. A draft of the legislation indicates that the plan would appropriate the sums 'necessary for payments for cost-sharing reductions' beginning in December 2017 and lasting through 2019." Despite this bipartisan effort to avoid the substantial adverse consequences of the loss of the CSR reimbursements, President Trump, as quoted in the article, tweeted in response, "I am supportive of Lamar as a person & also of the process, but I can never support bailing out ins co's who have made a fortune w/ O'Care." Sarah Huckabee Sanders, the White House press secretary, later confirmed that President Trump was in firm opposition to the effort by Senators Alexander and Murray to defuse the CSR crisis.

The dilemma facing insurance companies was that they were required to post their premiums for 2018 while the tumult of the CSR discussions was ongoing and before President Trump had announced his final decision whether to fund the CSRs for 2018. For a substantial number of insurers, the simplest way to avoid the coming confusion over CSRs and premiums was simply to exit the market. Crespin and DeLeire (2019) found that the number of insurance companies offering coverage on Healthcare.gov dropped from 232 in 2016 to 132 in 2018.

Corlette, Lucia, and Kona (2017) reported that "in 30 states, insurers assumed CSR payments would not be made, and concentrated the resulting premium increase onto marketplace silver plans only. Doing so maximizes that amount of premium subsidy consumers receive because the entire price increase is borne by silver plans on the marketplace. It also insulates unsubsidized consumers from the price increase if they purchase a plan outside the marketplace." They pointed out that 13 states made the same assumption but spread the premium increases across various combinations of plan levels, while only five states kept premiums largely unchanged on the assumption that the CSRs would be paid. (Data from insurers in two states were unavailable.)

In November, Rae, Levitt, and Semanskee (2017) used the differential premiums for bronze and silver level plans to estimate how many of those who remained uninsured could obtain a bronze-level health insurance plan either for free or for less than the tax penalty those who remained uninsured faced as a result of the ACA's individual mandate prior to the revocation of the penalty by Congress:

> We estimate that over half (54%) of the subsidy eligible–uninsured could purchase a bronze plan for 2018 for no premium contribution, after accounting for the premium subsidy. An additional 16% of this group could purchase a bronze plan for less than the cost of the tax penalty if they do not secure minimum essential coverage. Altogether 70% of subsidy eligible–uninsured (5.8 million people) are able to purchase a Bronze plan for nothing or less than the cost of the individual mandate penalty. (p. 3)

Branham and DeLeire (2019) compared the populations covered by a bronze-level plan in 2017 and in 2018, the first year in which the elevated silver-level premiums resulted in substantially increased PTCs. Of all those enrolling in coverage through a health exchange, 34.3% had a zero-premium bronze plan available to them in 2017, while 52.6% had such a plan available in 2018. As age is a factor in determining the premiums charged through the exchanges, a higher percentage of zero-premium plans were available to those aged 35 or older than to those younger than 35. Not all those eligible for a zero-premium plan elected to enroll in such a plan. Those with incomes between 100% and 250% of FPL needed to enroll in a silver-level plan in order to qualify for the CSRs.

It is also important to realize that the positive impact of the rising PTCs as a consequence of the silver-loading insurance companies used did not apply to individuals and families with incomes greater than 400% of FPL, as they were not eligible for PTCs. With rising premiums across all levels of coverage for those without PTCs, many of these people elected to drop their coverage rather than pay the increased premiums. The US Centers for Medicare & Medicaid Services (2019) analyzed enrollment trends in health insurance available through the exchanges for those eligible for PTCs and those ineligible. The report found that "average monthly enrollment across the entire individual market decreased by 7 percent nationally between 2017 and 2018 at the same time premiums increased by 26 percent." The report also indicated, "The decrease in enrollment between 2017 and 2018 occurred entirely among people who did not receive PTC subsidies." Among those ineligible for PTCs, enrollment declined by 24% between 2017 and 2018, while it increased by 4% for those eligible for PTCs. It seems clear that the political tug of war over funding the CSRs had its principal adverse impact on those with incomes high enough that they did not qualify for PTCs.

An analysis by Fehr, Cox, and Levitt (2019) found that, in the first quarter of 2019, enrollment in exchange plans eligible for PTCs increased slightly, while enrollment in ineligible plans dropped by about 7%. This decline was also seen in the private, off-exchange health insurance market, where no plans are eligible for PTCs. The authors pointed out two reasons for these declines: rising premiums and the end of the individual mandate tax penalty that resulted from the tax reform act passed in December 2017. I will discuss the many and complex impacts of the tax reform act in the following chapter.

While premiums increased substantially across nearly all states in 2018 for coverage purchased on the exchanges, once the insurance companies had reset their premiums to cover the loss of remuneration for the CSRs, there was little need for premium increases in the exchanges for the 2019 year. An analysis by Kamal, Cox, Long, and colleagues (2018) found that rates published by insurance companies for the 2019 enrollment period remained relatively flat, actually decreasing in a number of states. For the benchmark silver plan, rates increased in 24 states and the District of Columbia, decreased in 23 states, and were unchanged in three. Over all 50 states and the District of Columbia, the average change from 2018 to 2019 was a decrease of 0.5%. However, a separate analysis by Kamal, Cox, Fehr, and colleagues (2018) included plans sold off the ACA exchanges on the private health insurance market. As I will discuss in the following chapter, the Trump administration issued a series of regulatory changes that allowed policies that did not meet ACA coverage requirements to be sold in the private market. When these authors included off-exchange plans in their analysis, the overall average premium increased by 6%.

Aaron-Dine (2019) used a mathematical analysis to estimate the overall effects of the end of CSR payments to insurers and of the consequent silver loading on overall enrollment in exchange plans. Aaron-Dine concludes that "the administration's decision to end CSR payments has increased HealthCare.gov enrollment among PTC-eligible consumers by about 400,000 people. Extrapolating these results to state-based Marketplaces . . . implies a total increase of about 500,000, or about 5 percent." The irony of the Trump administration's decision, in concurrence with that of the Republican-led Congress, is that it has actually resulted in a substantial benefit to lower-income individuals and families, with significantly increased costs for the federal government.

The US Centers for Medicare & Medicaid Services (2019b) examined the changes in premium for coverage in 2020 issued by participating insurance plans. Looking at rates for a 27-year-old individual, it reported that rates across states participating in Healthcare.gov for the benchmark silver plan decreased by 4% as compared to rates for 2019. Assuming that the 27-year-old earns 150% of FPL, the average monthly premium in 2020 for the lowest-price silver plan, after taking PTCs into account, would be $52. By signing up for this plan, the individual would also be eligible for the CSRs mandated by the ACA. By contrast, a family of four with an income of 250% of FPL could purchase the lowest-price silver plan for $371 per month after applying the PTCs.

The US Centers for Medicare & Medicaid Services report (2019b) also found that the number of insurers offering plans on Healthcare.gov in 2020 increased from 155 to 175. This rebound is another sign that the initial adverse impacts on insurers of ending the CSR reimbursements had largely been ameliorated.

Fehr, Kamal, and Cox (2019) analyzed proposed premiums for 2020 for insurers on both Healthcare.gov and the individual state exchanges. They reported a very interesting finding, with substantial policy significance. A 40-year-old with an income of $25,000, equaling 200% of FPL, would, after taking PTCs into account, be eligible to purchase a bronze-level plan for zero premium in 55% of counties nationally. The unexpected finding is that the same individual would be eligible to purchase a gold-level plan for zero premium in 7% of counties nationally. Neither the bronze- nor the gold-level plan would qualify the individual for CSRs. As the authors describe, "Low-income consumers will need to consider whether it makes sense to purchase a metal level other than silver, as a lower premium plan may come with significantly higher deductibles, copays, or coinsurance." For someone who expects to need little medical care other than the preventive care services provided without cost to patients, it might make sense to accept a zero-premium plan rather than paying the substantially higher silver premium.

Congress Takes a Second Tack in Trying to Fiscally Disrupt Insurance Coverage under the ACA

When the ACA was passed in 2010, it created an entirely new market structure for insurance companies to compete to enroll the millions of people who were expected to obtain coverage. In addition, the ACA created a new form of health insurance plans: the nonprofit consumer cooperative plan. The goal was for every person enrolling in coverage to have a choice between a for-profit and a nonprofit plan.

From the perspective of the insurance companies, this new market structure created a potentially serious risk: "One concern with the guaranteed availability of insurance is that consumers who are most in need of health care may be more likely to purchase insurance. This phenomenon, known as adverse selection, can lead to higher average premiums, thereby disrupting the insurance market and undermining the goals of reform. Uncertainty about the health status of enrollees could also make insurers cautious about offering plans in a reformed individual market or cause them to be overly conservative in setting premiums" (Cox et al. 2016, p. 1).

Recognizing the uncertainty and the associated risks insurance companies faced when they elected to participate in the marketplace, the ACA created a plan for the federal government to provide back-up coverage to reimburse companies enrolling a disproportionate number of high-cost individuals in their plans. This coverage, known as reinsurance, was included in the ACA for the first three years of the new health insurance exchanges. The legislation referred to this three-year period as the "risk corridor."

As described by the Centers for Medicare & Medicaid Services, Center for Consumer Information and Insurance Oversight (2015):

> Section 1342 of the Affordable Care Act directs the Secretary of the Department of Health and Human Services (HHS) to establish a temporary risk corridors program that provides issuers of qualified health plans (QHPs) in the individual and small group markets additional protection against uncertainty in claims costs during the first three years of the Marketplace. The program . . . encourages issuers to keep their

rates stable as they adjust to the new health insurance reforms in the early years of the Marketplaces.

Cox and colleagues (2016, p. 10) have described the financial structure of these risk corridors: "The Risk Corridors program set a target for exchange participating insurers to spend 80% of premium dollars on health care and quality improvement. Insurers with costs less than 3% of the target amount must pay into the risk corridors program; the funds collected were used to reimburse plans with costs that exceed 3% of the target amount." Under the ACA, all insurance companies in the individual and small group market are expected to spend at least 80% of premiums collected on providing care to covered enrollees. This is why the risk corridors use the 80% level as the reference point.

A central policy aspect of the risk corridor payments was the assumption that the funds collected from those companies with lower than expected costs might be less than the funds owed to companies with higher than expected costs: "In the original statute, risk corridor payments were not required to net to zero, meaning that the federal government could experience an increase in revenues or an increase in costs under the program" (Cox et al. 2016, p. 11). This backup responsibility of the federal government was confirmed in a description of the risk corridor program issued by the Centers for Medicare & Medicaid Services, Center for Consumer Information and Insurance Oversight (2019): "The temporary risk corridors program protects qualified health plans from uncertainty in rate setting from 2014 to 2016 by having the Federal government share risk in losses and gains."

As described in chapter 4, in the elections of November 2014, Republicans increased their majority in the House of Representatives and took over leadership in the Senate. This gave the Republicans the ability to establish federal spending limits starting in the 2015 fiscal year, the first year in which risk corridor collections and reimbursements were to be made under the ACA: "Although the statute does not explicitly state that the amount paid to insurers cannot exceed the amount collected, Congress passed appropriations riders imposing such a requirement for 2014 and again for 2015" (Jost 2016b).

As a consequence of these appropriations riders, in November 2015, the Centers for Medicare & Medicaid Services, Center for Consumer Information and Insurance Oversight announced that aggregate risk corridor gains were $362 million while aggregate risk corridor losses were $2.87 billion. Based on these numbers, those insurance companies who exceeded the 3% loss in 2014 would be paid only 12.6% of that loss. "Risk corridors were intended to reduce overall financial uncertainty for insurers, though they largely did not fulfill that goal following congressional changes to the program" (Cox et al., p. 12).

The Centers for Medicare & Medicaid Services, Center for Consumer Information and Insurance Oversight (2016a) announced the repayment rates for risk corridor losses incurred during 2015. "Today, we are confirming that all 2015 benefit year risk corridors collections will be used to pay a portion of balances on 2014 benefit year risk corridors payments." This meant that there would be no funds available to reimburse insurers who exceeded the risk corridor loss threshold for 2015. The same thing happened for 2016, the final year of the risk corridor program under the ACA. The losses incurred in 2016 were simply added to the unpaid losses from 2015, and any risk corridor revenues collected were again applied to the outstanding losses from 2014. As Jost (2018) reported, "On November 13, CMS announced results for the risk corridor program for 2016. Government obligations to insurers grew by almost $4 billion while collections came to only $27 million. The 2016 collections will be applied to 2014 obligations, but unless insurers prevail in the three dozen lawsuits currently pending in the federal court of claims, they will never recover the whole $12 billion they are owed under the program."

As a consequence of the appropriations riders Republicans in Congress had imposed on the risk corridor program, insurance companies incurred billions of dollars of losses for which they would not be reimbursed. As reported by Bagley (2016, p. 2018), "The inability to make full risk-corridor payments devastated some insurers. Hit particularly hard were the new cooperative health plans, which were established with the support of generous ACA loans." By the end of 2020, only 3 of the 26 original co-ops were still in business (Galewitz 2020). The nonprofit health insurance co-ops were a core element in creating and maintaining competitive health insurance exchanges across the country. "The loss of the co-ops, together with the withdrawal of several large insurers from a number of states, has led to a sharp reduction in competition on the exchanges" (Bagley 2016, p. 2018).

When it became apparent that there would be no appropriated funds to pay risk corridor losses for 2015, in September 2016 the secretary of Health and Human Services under the Obama administration made an announcement (Centers for Medicare & Medicaid Services, Center for Consumer Information and Insurance Oversight 2016b): "HHS recognizes that the Affordable Care Act requires the Secretary to make full payments to issuers. HHS will record risk corridors payments due as an obligation of the United States Government for which full payment is required." Jost (2016b) reported the response of congressional Republicans to this statement: "This statement brought forth a storm of criticism from Republican members of Congress, who held a hearing on the issue and sent a number of letters to HHS Secretary Burwell expressing concern that HHS might be attempting to circumvent the limits Congress had placed on appropriations by settling the cases using money from the judgment fund, which funds judgments and settlements in Court of Claims cases." It seemed increasingly clear that insurance companies who had relied on the risk corridor payments when setting their premium rates were not going to get those payments unless they took legal action against the government.

Bagley (2016, p. 2018) reported, "Health insurers struck back. In February 2016, a failed Oregon co-op filed a class-action lawsuit to recover what it was owed under the risk-corridor program. At least seven other lawsuits seeking reimbursement have since been filed." However, these suits were filed shortly before the November 2016 elections. While the Obama administration had expressed an openness to discussing a possible settlement to these lawsuits, once President Trump had taken office, the Justice Department contested these suits vigorously.

Jost (2017c) described the court's response to the suit: "On January 3, 2017, Judge Margaret Sweeney of the United States Court of Claims certified Health Republic Insurance Company v. United States as a class action. This is one of more than a dozen cases that have been brought by insurers in the Court of Claims challenging the failure of the government to pay marketplace insurers amounts that they claim were due to them under the ACA's risk corridor program."

One of these suits was brought by Land of Lincoln Health, a health insurance co-op that was bankrupted by the failure to recoup about $73 million in losses under the risk corridor. In November 2016, the federal judge hearing the case dismissed the suit, ruling against Land of Lincoln, which subsequently filed an appeal. Moda Health Plan, a private company offering health insurance in Oregon, Alaska, and Washington, sued to recover about $214 million in unpaid risk corridors payments for 2014 and 2015. In February 2017, a different judge granted a partial summary judgment in favor of Moda Health Plan. The Justice Department appealed that ruling (Keith 2018).

"In January 2018, the Federal Circuit heard oral arguments in Land of Lincoln and Moda . . . On June 14, 2018, a three-judge panel of the Court of Appeals for the Federal Circuit issued an opinion in Moda Health Plan v. United States. By a 2-1 majority, the appellate panel concluded that the government does not have to pay health insurers that offered qualified health plans (QHPs) the full amount owed to them in risk corridors payments." By issuing that ruling, the appeals court also upheld the earlier decision against Land of Lincoln. As Keith (2018) concluded, "For now, insurers cannot recover the more than $12 billion owed in outstanding risk corridors payments."

Both insurers appealed this decision to the Supreme Court. As Keith (2019b) has reported, "In late June 2019 the Supreme Court agreed to hear the insurers' appeal during its next term." Jost (2019) subsequently reported that the cases of Moda and Land of Lincoln will be combined with two other cases, and "the Supreme Court will hear oral arguments in lawsuits brought by four health insurers seeking damages against the United States for its failure to fully pay risk-corridor payments promised by the Affordable Care Act (ACA)." The court's decision would likely affect the dozens of outstanding lawsuits against the government, including a class action suit with about 150 claimants.

The Supreme Court heard oral arguments on these cases on December 10. As reported in the *New York Times*, "The Supreme Court seemed inclined on Tuesday to require the federal government to live up to its promise to shield insurance companies from some of the risks they took in participating in the exchanges established by President Barack Obama's health care law, the Affordable Care Act" (Liptak 2019). Phil Galewitz (2019), reporting for *Kaiser Health News*, had a similar impression of the court's response: "During the hour of oral arguments, six justices appeared to favor the insurers' argument . . . A ruling on the case, *Maine Community Health Options v. United States*, is expected in the spring."

The Supreme Court issued its ruling on April 27, 2020. The ruling had consolidated three earlier cases: *Maine Community Health Options v. United States*, *Moda Health Plan Inc. v. United States*, and *Land of Lincoln Mutual Health Insurance Co. v. United States*. As reported by Adam Liptak in the *New York Times* (2020), "The Supreme Court ruled Monday that the federal government must live up to its promise to shield insurance companies from some of the risks they took in participating in the exchanges established by President Barack Obama's health care law, the Affordable Care Act. Justice Sonia Sotomayor, writing for the majority in the 8-to-1 ruling, said the court's decision vindicated 'a principle as old as the nation itself: The government should honor its obligations.'" Liptak goes on to quote Justice Sotomayor's concluding remarks: "In sum, the plain terms of the risk corridors provision created an obligation neither contingent on nor limited by the availability of appropriations or other funds."

As a result of the court's ruling, the federal government is required to pay the involved insurance companies a total of $12.2 billion. For those co-ops that went out of business, these funds will help to pay down their debts.

The Courts also Consider Cost-Sharing Reductions

While this chapter has focused most of its attention on the legal challenges to the risk corridor payments, another set of lawsuits was pursued in parallel: "Insurers have sued HHS for at least $2.3 billion in unpaid cost-sharing reduction payments (CSRs) since the Trump administration decided to stop making the payments in October 2017. To date, six insurers—in front of three different judges at the Court of Federal Claims—have succeeded in their challenges over unpaid CSRs" (Keith 2019c). Keith goes on to point out that "three of the cases—brought by Montana Health CO-OP, Sanford Health Plan, and Community Health Choice—have already been appealed to the Federal Circuit and were consolidated." Nine other cases involving unpaid CSRs are pending in lower courts.

Keith (2019d) provided an update on these lawsuits: "On October 22, 2019, Judge Margaret M. Sweeney issued a final decision in a class action lawsuit brought by insurers over unpaid cost-sharing reduction (CSR) payments. She held that the estimated 100 insurers in the class are owed nearly $1.6 billion in unpaid CSRs for 2017 and 2018." On January 9, 2020, the Court of Appeals for the Federal Circuit in Washington, DC, heard oral arguments in the appeal of Judge Sweeny's ruling. The appeal consolidated the three cases mentioned above with the suit filed by Maine Community Health Options.

The issues raised in the CSR cases are similar to those raised in the risk corridor suit. Following the Supreme Court's ruling in the risk corridor cases, Keith (2020a) concluded that "the Supreme Court's ruling bolsters the conclusion that insurers are entitled to unpaid CSRs. The CSR statute is a 'shall pay' statute that, like Section 1342, could be viewed as creating a government obligation even in the absence of an explicit appropriation."

Consistent with this perspective, on August 14, 2020, the Court of Appeals for the Federal Circuit issued its ruling. As Keith (2020b) reports, "The Federal Circuit agreed with the lower courts that Section 1402 imposes an 'unambiguous obligation' on the government to make CSR payments to insurers and that this obligation is enforceable for damages in court." The court ruled that the insurance companies who brought the suit are entitled to full payment of the CSR costs incurred in 2017. For 2018 and beyond, the amount the companies are due will need to be reduced by the amount of the increased premium tax credits they received as a consequence of silver loading. The court of appeals remanded the cases to the lower courts to determine the amount due for the later years.

Jost (2020) raises an important point that remains unresolved following the ruling. "The decisions raise as many questions as they resolve. They do not require the government to resume CSR payments unless Congress appropriates the money but do allow for insurers to recover their losses if the government does not make the payments." It remains to be seen whether Congress will elect to end this controversy by authorizing the CSR payments required under the ACA or whether the payments will be handled by the courts.

SEVEN

Continuing Efforts to Weaken
the Affordable Care Act

AS I have addressed in the previous chapters, following the passage of the Affordable Care Act in 2010, the Republican forces in both the House of Representatives and the Senate have been united in an effort to undo the act. During the final years of the Obama administration, Congress passed legislation that would have either repealed or revamped major portions of the ACA. Not surprisingly, President Obama vetoed it.

With the election of President Trump in 2016 and the strong Republican majorities in both houses of Congress, the repeal process gained new momentum. In May 2017, the House of Representatives passed the American Health Care Act, which would have repealed key portions of the ACA through the reconciliation process. When the repeal legislation moved on to the Senate, the Republican leadership there elected to pursue a secretive review and amendment process, carried on largely behind closed doors.

Based on this process, Senate majority leader Mitch McConnell elected to introduce a substantially revised bill, renamed the Better Care Reconciliation Act. When McConnell was unable to garner sufficient support among Republicans in the Senate for that bill, he introduced a watered-down version, the Health Care Freedom Act, or "skinny repeal." When that bill came up for a final vote, it was defeated with 51 senators voting against and 49 in favor. Three Republicans—Susan Collins, Lisa Murkowski, and John McCain—joined Democrats in voting against the bill. In one final attempt to repeal parts of the ACA, Republican senators Lindsey Graham of South Carolina and Bill Cassidy of Louisiana submitted a bill to repeal core elements of the ACA. When Senator McConnell realized that he still did not have the Republican votes to pass the bill, he simply let it drop, without ever having a formal vote.

In light of their failure to attain repeal of the ACA, congressional Republicans then attempted to destabilize the financing for the ACA through two principal means. Under the Obama administration, the House of Representatives had filed a lawsuit to prohibit the administration's reimbursement of insurance companies for the added financial burden of the cost sharing reductions. As discussed in the previous chapter, once President Trump was elected, he chose to accept the House's limitations through settling the lawsuit.

Even though they were not going to receive reimbursements for them, insurance companies still had to grant enrollees the CSRs mandated by the ACA. For coverage through the ACA exchanges in 2018, the failure to make the CSR reimbursements led to major increases in premiums for those enrolling in a silver-tier plan. However, since more than 80% of those enrolling in exchange coverage were eligible for premium tax credits that capped the amount of premiums they had to pay, most people paid either the same premium or a reduced premium for coverage. Those not eligible for PTCs were able to enroll in either a bronze or gold plan, thus avoiding the increased premiums assigned to silver plans. The end result was substantially increased costs for the federal government with only a minimal adverse impact on those purchasing coverage through the exchanges.

Republicans in the House tried a second means to fiscally destabilize the ACA. Again as discussed in the previous chapter, the original legislation provided three years of backup coverage that would reimburse insurance companies whose plans enrolled a disproportionate number of high-cost individuals. This reinsurance program was referred to as risk corridors. The House imposed a requirement that the risk corridor payments be revenue neutral. This meant that the payments to those companies that had enrolled a disproportionate number of sicker, high-cost individuals had to be made out of the refunds paid by those companies that had enrolled a lower number. During the first year of coverage, the promised risk corridor payments were substantially greater than the refunds. As a consequence, those companies that experienced a substantial loss in 2014, the first year of coverage, were paid only 12.6% of that loss. By the end of the three-year risk corridor period, billions of dollars in unpaid costs remained, leading to the bankruptcy of a number of insurance companies, especially the nonprofit co-op plans the ACA had helped to create. Many other companies simply left the market. Those companies that had unreimbursed losses under the risk corridor plan subsequently filed lawsuits in federal court to recoup their losses. The Supreme Court heard appeals from those lawsuits in December 2019 and in April 2020 issued its ruling in favor of the plaintiffs. In August 2020 the Court of Appeals for the Federal Circuit issued a similar ruling regarding the payment to insurance companies of the costs associated with the CSRs.

Despite these efforts to destabilize the ACA marketplaces, by 2019, exchange premiums had largely stabilized, with historically low increases. In light of these failures either to repeal the ACA or to destabilize its financial base, President Trump in concert with congressional Republicans made a series of attempts to weaken the ACA through other, more focused changes.

The Repeal of the Individual Mandate Tax Penalty

As I describe in my *U.S. Health Policy* textbook (Barr 2016, p. 13), the "ACA includes a provision known commonly as the individual mandate that requires most people in the United States to maintain a minimum level of health insurance coverage for themselves and their dependents . . . [T]hose who fail to maintain this coverage will be required to pay a penalty to the federal government. The penalty will be collected as part of the individual's yearly income tax return." A group of private businesses filed a lawsuit, *National Federation of Independent Business v. Sebelius*, challenging the individual mandate, arguing that individual choices in matters such as the acquisition of health insurance were not part of interstate commerce, and the law was therefore in violation of Article 1 Section 8 of the US Constitution, the interstate commerce clause.

The Supreme Court heard the final appeal of the case and issued its ruling in June 2012. "The Court upheld the individual mandate . . . [T]he Court agreed that the interstate commerce clause of Article 1, Section 8, did not apply to the decision to purchase health insurance, as individual decisions of this type are not part of interstate commerce. However, while the federal government may not force someone to acquire health insurance, it can levy an extra tax on those who elect not to obtain coverage . . . under the federal government's authority under Article 1, Section 8, to 'lay and collect taxes'" (Barr 2016, p. 14).

What, though, if Congress were to remove the tax penalty but keep in place the mandate to purchase health insurance? Since the mandate to purchase insurance itself was not permitted under the Constitution but applying the tax penalty was, would removal of the tax penalty, leaving the mandate in place, cause this portion of the ACA to violate the Constitution? If that were found to be the case, would that constitutional violation then invalidate the entire ACA? Congress was betting that it would and elected to take this tack, with the support of the Trump administration.

Recall that the Republican efforts to repeal the ACA faltered and ultimately failed in September 2017, as the federal fiscal year came to a close. Congress had elected to use the reconciliation process in its attempt to repeal the ACA, and authorization for a reconciliation bill expires at the end of the fiscal year. As of October 1, 2017, Congress had the option of authorizing a new reconciliation process for the new fiscal year. However, "on October 1st, the federal fiscal year (FY) 2017 came to an end and with it the authorization to use the budget reconciliation process to pass ACA repeal legislation as well . . . But for FY 18, the priority for the Administration and Congress was tax reform, and there can only be one budget reconciliation bill per year" (Frommer 2018).

President Trump had set tax reform as his top priority for the new fiscal year. Accordingly, the first action the Republican House took in the new fiscal year was, on November 2, to introduce the Tax Cuts and Jobs Act as H.R. 1 (2017–2018). Although its main focus was to substantially reduce tax rates, especially on high-income taxpayers and certain businesses, the bill also included a section that amended the tax law to revoke the tax penalty that was in place to enforce the individual mandate to purchase health insurance. Effective in 2019 taxpayers were no longer required to provide documentation that they had had insurance coverage in filing their 2018 taxes.

In November 2017, the Congressional Budget Office (2017) issued a report that estimated the effects of repealing the individual mandate tax penalty, key among which were the following:

- Federal budget deficits would be reduced by about $338 billion between 2018 and 2027.
- The number of people with health insurance would decrease by 4 million in 2019 and 13 million in 2027.
- Average premiums in the nongroup market would increase by about 10% in most years of the decade.

The principal reason for the expected decrease in enrollment and increase in premiums was that, absent the tax penalty of the mandate, people who were younger and relatively healthy would be most likely to drop their health insurance coverage, leaving as a greater percentage of the market those who are sicker, with higher expected costs. Beyond these projections, the CBO also concluded that, "in that baseline, the ACA's other provisions, including premium tax credits and cost-sharing reduction (CSR) subsidies in the marketplaces that the legislation established, are assumed to remain in place" (pp. 1–3).

In October both the House and the Senate passed budget resolutions authorizing the reconciliation process for the tax bill. H.R. 1 was referred to the House Ways and Means Committee, which issued its report on November 13, adding some amendments to the original bill. On November 16, the full House passed the tax bill by a vote of

227-205. All votes in favor were by Republicans, while 13 Republicans joined 192 Democrats in voting against the bill (2 Democrats did not submit votes).

The bill then went to the Senate Finance Committee, which amended the House version to include the revocation of the individual mandate tax penalty. That was the only part of the tax bill that addressed the ACA. By December 2, the Senate had completed its discussion of the bill, and passed it on December 2 by a vote of 51-49. Republican senator Bob Corker of Tennessee joined all 48 Democrats in voting against the bill, with all of the remaining 51 Republicans voting in favor. A House-Senate conference committee met to reconcile the differences between the two bills, using the Senate's as the final version. On December 20, the House passed this final version by a vote of 224-201.

After passage of the final bill and Trump's signature, Frommer (2018) reported that "President Trump has described the repeal of the individual mandate enforcement provisions as tantamount to repeal of the ACA." Jost (2018, p. 13) reflected on what the repeal of the individual mandate might mean for the rest of the ACA: "The Senate has two reasons for repealing the individual mandate. First, and probably most important, the Joint Committee on Taxation scored the repeal as saving the federal government $318 billion over ten years. This gave Senate Republicans money they badly needed to increase tax cuts, including a permanent reduction in the corporate tax rate. The second reason, of course, was to follow through on the promise made to repeal at least part of the ACA."

Drew Altman of the Kaiser Family Foundation (2017) cited a series of public opinion polls regarding the revocation of the individual mandate. When asked about the mandate repeal itself, a minority of 42% of respondents were opposed. Altman then provided respondents with some additional information about the repeal and got the following results:

- When people learn that they will not be affected by the mandate if they already get insurance from their employer or from Medicare or Medicaid, 62% oppose eliminating it.

- When people are told that eliminating the mandate would increase premiums for people who buy their own coverage, as the CBO says it will, they also flip, with 60% opposing eliminating the mandate.

It appears the general public understood very little about what the mandate repeal might mean for them.

In April, the Kaiser Family Foundation (2018) also published the results of a public opinion poll about the impact of the individual mandate revocation. "The survey also finds a lack of awareness about the status of the mandate penalty, with 1 in 5 non-group enrollees (19%) saying they are aware the penalty has been repealed but is still in effect for this year. The mandate continues to rank far down on a list of 'major reasons' people give for buying their own insurance in 2018." The authors reported that "the survey also finds that about half of the public say they believe the ACA marketplaces are 'collapsing.'"

The Kaiser Family Foundation (2019) analyzed enrollment in the individual health insurance market nationally and found that "overall enrollment in the individual market fell 5% to 13.7 million in the first quarter of 2019 following the repeal of the Affordable Care Act's individual mandate penalty." The decrease was mostly among those who had previously acquired their coverage outside of the exchanges, through private brokers or directly from the insurance companies. The encouragement of noncompliant health insurance plans, discussed in the next section, may also have contributed to the decline.

The Expansion of Health Insurance
That Does Not Comply with ACA Regulations

Recall from chapter 5 that on the January 20, 2017, the day he was inaugurated, President Trump issued Executive Order Number 13765, in which he stated explicitly, "It is the policy of my Administration to seek the prompt repeal of the Patient Protection and Affordable Care Act (Public Law 111-148), as amended." By October 2017, it was clear that efforts in Congress to repeal all or part of the ACA had failed. Accordingly, on October 12, 2017, President Trump issued a new executive order.

Executive Order 13813 was titled "Presidential Executive Order Promoting Healthcare Choice and Competition across the United States." (Trump 2017b). The order states:

> The Patient Protection and Affordable Care Act (PPACA), however, has severely limited the choice of healthcare options available to many Americans and has produced large premium increases in many State individual markets for health insurance . . . The PPACA has also largely failed to provide meaningful choice or competition between insurers . . . my Administration will prioritize three areas for improvement in the near term: association health plans (AHPs), short-term, limited-duration insurance (STLDI), and health reimbursement arrangements (HRAs).
>
> (i) Expanding access to AHPs can help small businesses overcome this competitive disadvantage by allowing them to group together to self-insure or purchase large group health insurance. Expanding access to AHPs will also allow more small businesses to avoid many of the PPACA's costly requirements.
>
> (ii) STLDI is exempt from the onerous and expensive insurance mandates and regulations included in title I of the PPACA. This can make it an appealing and affordable alternative to government-run exchanges for many people without coverage available to them through their workplaces.
>
> (iii) Expanding the flexibility and use of HRAs would provide many Americans, including employees who work at small businesses, with more options for financing their healthcare.

The order then goes on to grant specific governmental agencies the authority to enact or enable these alternative health plan arrangements, which had not previously been authorized under the ACA.

Pollitz and Claxton (2018) described the new types of health plans that would be permissible under President Trump's executive order. Association health plans (AHPs) "would permit small employers and self-employed individuals to buy a new type of association health plan coverage that does not have to meet all requirements applicable to other ACA-compliant small group and non-group health plans." In essence, groups of small employers or individuals who otherwise have no business connection would band together to negotiate with a health insurance company to offer coverage to them as if they were a large employer. Accordingly, they would not be subject to many of the requirements for insurance sold to individuals through the exchanges. For example, they would not be required to cover all essential health benefits. They could also vary their premiums without the limits based on age differentials, gender, and geography that are part of the ACA. "As a result, AHPs could provide self-employed individuals an alternative to individual health insurance that provides fewer benefits with more rating flexibility. As nearly one-third (31%) of individual market enrollees are self-employed, the impact of AHPs could be significant" (p. 6).

The authors also describe the new regulations "that would promote the sale of short-term, limited duration [STLD] health insurance policies that offer less expensive coverage because they are not subject to ACA market rules" (Pollitz and Claxton 2018, p. 3). These policies would offer a level of benefits that is substantially less than that of ACA compliant plans. Pollitz and colleagues (2018) identified the following limitations of STLD policies as compared to ACA-compliant policies:

- Often medically underwritten—applicants with health conditions can be turned down or charged higher premiums, without limit, based on health status, gender, age, and other factors
- Exclude coverage for pre-existing conditions
- Not required to cover essential health benefits
- May impose lifetime and annual limits
- Not subject to cost sharing limits
- Not constrained by other ACA market requirements

It should be clear that the level of coverage provided by STLD policies is substantially less than ACA policies. In addition, they do not guarantee the option to renew the policy after its period of coverage. If a person on such a policy were to develop a serious illness, they would likely be unable to renew the policy upon its expiration.

Under the Obama administration, STLD policies were permitted for a maximum of 3 months of coverage. Under the individual mandate rules, those who lose their coverage by loss of employment could enroll in a

3-month STLD policy and be exempt from the mandate penalty. "In February of this year [2018], the Trump Administration published a proposed regulation amending the definition of short-term policies to include those offering a maximum coverage period of less than 12 months" (Pollitz et al. 2018, p. 4). The authors go on to express their concern about the potential adverse impacts of this expansion of STLD policies. "The combined effect of repealing the individual mandate penalty and the administration's efforts to promote the sale of short-term plans could result in fewer people signing up for ACA-compliant plans and higher premiums in the ACA-compliant individual market, potentially adversely affecting the stability of the ACA-compliant individual market" (p. 8).

Keith (2018) reported that the final rule issued by the Department of Health and Human Services governing STLD plans allows them to be sold for up to 364 days of coverage. The rule also allows plans to be renewed up to a total of 36 months. Keith reports that "new short-term plans are expected to attract healthy enrollees, which will have the effect of increasing premiums for those who remain in the ACA Marketplaces. The agencies estimate that this will result in higher federal outlays for premium subsidies of about $28.2 billion during the period 2019–28" (p. 1544). The agencies also predicted that enrollment in STLDs will grow by 1.4 million, with a corresponding decrease of 1.3 million enrollees in the ACA exchange market.

By October 2018, insurance companies had posted their premiums for ACA coverage in 2019. Kamal and colleagues (2018) estimated the impact of the expansion of STLDs in combination with repeal of the individual mandate on premiums. The authors "found that 2019 premiums will be an average of 6% higher, as a direct result of individual mandate repeal and expansion of more loosely regulated plans, than would otherwise be the case" (p. 1). However, in some areas of the country, silver-level premiums were decreasing for 2019 because of the overly cautious silver loading of premiums for 2018 triggered by the end of the CSR reimbursement. These decreasing premiums may offset the increase identified by this study.

Goe (2019) has identified a further weakness of STLD plans that many consumers may not be aware of. In addition to their coverage limitations, "another problem with these health plans is that they do not offer a network of health providers, which leads to unexpected 'balance bills' for the consumer." Balance billing occurs when a patient receives care from a physician or other provider who is not in the contracted network of providers for the plan. The plan will pay the amount agreed to by providers in the network, which is often substantially less than the typical out-of-network charge. The patient is then responsible for the balance. Very often patients are unaware that the provider they are seeing is not within their insurance company's contracted network. The often substantial balance bills they receive are often a complete surprise to them.

Seervai, Gunja, and Collins (2019) recounted the experience of a patient who encountered just such a surprise. Francesca Nuñez had lost her job and the health insurance that went with it. She signed up for a non-ACA-compliant plan that had a monthly premium of only $245. She went to her regular doctor, whom she had been seeing for 14 years under her old insurance, for a routine annual checkup. Shortly after her visit, she received a bill from the doctor for $300. "Nuñez was shocked. Having recently lost her regular income, she could scarcely afford the bill. She paid it, but subsequently cancelled the coverage, joining the ranks of the 30 million Americans who are uninsured." Based on this story, the authors concluded, "Non-ACA-compliant plans are offered outside the ACA marketplaces and may seem attractive because they are cheaper. But, like many plans prior to the ACA, many leave people at risk of high medical bills because of hidden costs and limited coverage."

The Expansion of Health Reimbursement Arrangements (HRAs)

The third change made by President Trump's Executive Order was to expand the circumstances in which health reimbursement arrangements (HRAs) may be used to pay medical bills. HRAs are plans under which employees can set aside pretax funds from their own earnings, which they can then tap into to pay out-of-pocket health care costs. Originally, HRA funds could not be used to pay health insurance premiums. As described by the US Centers for Medicare & Medicaid Services (n.d.), "New rules released by the Departments of Labor, Health and Human Services, and the Treasury permit employers to offer a new 'individual coverage HRA' as an alternative to traditional group health plan coverage . . . [I]ndividual coverage HRAs can be used to reimburse premiums for individual health insurance chosen by the employee."

When the final rules were published in June 2019, Keith (2019a) reported that "the HRA rule completes the regulatory trifecta from President Trump's executive order in October 2017." HRAs had previously been available to assist employees in enrolling in the group health plan offered by the employer. "HRAs qualify for pre-tax treatment because they are considered group health plans. As group health plans, HRAs have historically not been able to be used to pay premiums for coverage in the individual market."

By providing employees with tax-free funds to pay premiums for health insurance obtained outside the workplace, this new policy in effect encourages certain employers to direct their employees to the private insurance market to obtain individual or family coverage. However, employees who use the HRA to acquire individual coverage are not also eligible for PTCs to subsidize their premiums. Also, under the new rules, employers cannot offer both an HRA and its traditional group coverage to the same group of employees. The employer may offer group coverage to full-time employees and HRA coverage to part-time employees. HRAs are also attractive to smaller employers who have less access to competitively priced group coverage for their employees.

Volk and Lucia (2019) assessed the potential market impacts of the new HRA arrangements: "This change could shift individuals from employer-based coverage, which insures more than half of all Americans under age 65, to the state-regulated individual markets, including the Affordable Care Act (ACA) marketplaces . . . Health care costs for these individuals would shift, in part, from employers to taxpayers and employees, who could end up with less-comprehensive coverage."

Keith reports that the Trump administration predicted that "an estimated 11.4 million people will be in an HRA-IIHIC [integrated with individual health insurance coverage] in 2029 while the number of people with traditional group health plan coverage will drop by up to 6.9 million." The administration also predicted that HRAs would increase premiums in the individual market, "because employers that will be attracted to the HRA option are expected to have slightly higher health care expenses than other employers and current individual market enrollees." HRAs appear to have the potential to disrupt the decades-old employer group health insurance model.

Reduced Funding for Navigator Enrollment Assistance Further Destabilizes ACA Markets

A key part of the ACA that has greatly facilitated enrollment in either ACA or in Medicaid or CHIP has been the enrollment navigator program. As described on Healthcare.gov (n.d.), a navigator is "an individual or organization that's trained and able to help consumers, small businesses, and their employees as they look for health coverage options through the Marketplace, including completing eligibility and enrollment forms. These individuals and organizations are required to be unbiased. Their services are free to consumers."

As described by Pollitz, Tolbert, and Diaz (2019), "The Affordable Care Act (ACA) created Navigator programs to provide outreach, education, and enrollment assistance to consumers eligible for marketplace and Medicaid coverage and requires that they be funded by the marketplaces." While states such as California that operate their own ACA exchange will typically fund the navigator program in the state, states that use Healthcare.gov rely on federal grants.

In 2016, the Centers for Medicare & Medicaid Services provided $63 million in funding for navigators in those states (Pollitz, Tolbert, and Diaz 2019). Following the election of President Trump "in 2017, however, CMS reduced federal Navigator funding to $36.1 million, then reduced funding again in 2018 to $10 million. The Trump administration has also reduced funding for outreach outside of navigator programs by 90%." Funding in 2019 was also capped at $10 million, a reduction of 84% from funding under the Obama administration. With this reduction, in many states navigators are able to provide assistance only through phone consultation or a website. In four states, the online navigator had no physical presence.

The Trump administration has encouraged private insurance brokers to take the place of navigators. As they rely on commissions from enrolling clients in coverage, "brokers were significantly less likely than Navigators to help individuals who were uninsured, had limited English proficiency, or who lacked internet at home. Brokers were also far less likely to help complete applications for Medicaid or CHIP for low-income consumers" (Pollitz, Tolbert, and Diaz 2019). These same brokers can earn their commissions by steering people to noncompliant plans such as STLD. Many who enroll in these plans are not aware of the plans' limitations, as described earlier in this chapter.

Attempts to Block Contraceptive Coverage for Women

When it was originally passed, the ACA included a requirement that those providing insurance under the ACA include as a covered benefit a range of preventive services at no cost to the patient. The section titled "Coverage of Certain Preventive Services Under the Affordable Care Act," includes the following:

> With respect to women, preventive care and screenings provided for in comprehensive guidelines supported by HRSA (not otherwise addressed by the recommendations of the Task Force), including all Food and Drug Administration (FDA)-approved contraceptives, sterilization procedures, and patient education and counseling for women with reproductive capacity, as prescribed by a health care provider (collectively, contraceptive services). (*Federal Register* 2015)

The ACA includes an important exception. The final regulations for Section 2713 "provided HRSA with the authority to exempt group health plans established or maintained by certain religious employers (and group health insurance coverage provided in connection with those plans) from the requirement to cover contraceptive services." The ACA allows religious employers, such as churches or religious schools, to provide health insurance without contraceptive coverage. Instead, the insurance company that offers this coverage to employers must provide a supplemental benefit, fully separate and distinct from the employer policy, that covers contraception at no cost to the employee. In this manner, the regulations respect the religious beliefs of the employer while also protecting employees.

On May 4, 2017, President Trump issued yet another executive order, this one instructing his administration to weaken a central element of the ACA (Trump 2017a). Executive Order 13798 is titled "Promoting Free Speech and Religious Liberty." Section 1 of the order states, "It shall be the policy of the executive branch to vigorously enforce Federal law's robust protections for religious freedom."

Section 2 requires that "the Department of the Treasury does not take any adverse action against any individual, house of worship, or other religious organization on the basis that such individual or organization speaks or has spoken about moral or political issues from a religious perspective." Section 3 then states, "The Secretary of the Treasury, the Secretary of Labor, and the Secretary of Health and Human Services shall consider issuing amended regulations, consistent with applicable law, to address conscience-based objections to the preventive-care mandate" (Trump 2017a). "Conscience-based objections" can be either religious or moral in nature.

What this order effectively does is to expand the range of employers exempted from providing contraception to employees to include "any individual, house of worship, or other religious organization" that objects to the provision of contraception to women. The new rule also removes the requirement that the company providing health insurance to an objecting employer provide contraception as a supplemental benefit to women. All the employer is required to do is to inform the insurance company of its religious objection, and contraceptive coverage is removed as a benefit under the employer's plan.

In October 2017, the Commonwealth of Pennsylvania filed a lawsuit in the District Court for its Eastern District, challenging these new Trump administration rules. "Today, December 15 . . . Judge Wendy Beetlestone of the federal district court for the Eastern District of Pennsylvania entered a preliminary injunction in the case of Pennsylvania v.

Trump. The injunction blocks the Trump administration from implementing its interim final rules providing for both religious and moral exemptions and accommodations from the contraceptive coverage requirement imposed under the Affordable Care Act's preventive services coverage requirement" (Jost 2017a).

The State of California filed a similar lawsuit in its District Court. California was joined by 12 other states and the District of Columbia. "On December 21, 2017, Judge Haywood Gilliam of the United States District Court for the Northern District of California entered a nationwide preliminary injunction in California v. Trump. The injunction blocks the Trump administration from implementing its interim final rules providing for religious and moral exemptions from the contraceptive coverage mandate imposed under the Affordable Care Act's preventive services coverage requirement" (Jost 2017b).

The Trump administration quickly appealed both cases. The Pennsylvania case was heard by the Third Circuit Court of Appeals, which issued its ruling on July 12, 2019, upholding the decision of the district court. The California case was heard by the Ninth Circuit Court of Appeals in San Francisco, which issued its ruling on October 22, 2019, also upholding the ruling of the District Court, blocking the Trump administration's expansion of the religious exemption. "While the Ninth Circuit ruling applies only to the plaintiff states, the Third Circuit upheld a lower court's preliminary nationwide injunction. This blocked the Trump administration from enforcing its new rules in all 50 states and DC" (Keith 2019b).

The Trump administration appealed the Third Circuit Court's ruling to the Supreme Court. A separate appeal to the Supreme Court was filed by the Little Sisters of the Poor, a religious organization described on its website as "an international congregation of Roman Catholic women" whose "mission is to offer the neediest elderly of every race and religion a home" (n.d.). The Supreme Court heard oral arguments in both cases on May 6, 2020. As described in the *New York Times* by Adam Liptak (2020a), "Even as the justices appeared deeply divided along the usual lines on Wednesday, there was broad agreement that the case, Little Sisters of the Poor v. Pennsylvania, No. 19–431, required the court to balance religious freedom against women's health." As reported separately by Keith (2020), "In the middle of the spectrum, Chief Justice Roberts and Justice Kagan seemed sympathetic to the idea that the federal government has the authority to create exemptions to the mandate, but that the current rules fail to balance the interests of religious liberty and women's access to contraceptives." Chief Justice John Roberts also expressed frustration that the court was having to consider these issues for the third time. Keith quotes him as saying, "The problem is that neither side in this debate wants the accommodation to work . . . [I]s it really the case that there is no way to resolve those differences?"

On July 9, 2020, according to Adam Liptak (2020b) in the *New York Times*, "The Supreme Court on Wednesday upheld a Trump administration regulation that lets employers with religious or moral objections limit women's access to birth control coverage under the Affordable Care Act. As a consequence of the ruling, about 70,000 to 126,000 women could lose contraceptive coverage from their employers, according to government estimates." The vote was 7-2, with Justices Sonia Sotomayor and Ruth Ginsburg objecting. It remains to be seen how this policy of the Trump administration will be impacted by the 2020 elections.

Legal Action to Block Association Health Plans

When President Trump announced his new policies to enable AHPs, many states were concerned that such plans could weaken and destabilize their health insurance markets. Accordingly, as announced on July 27, 2018 by Morse (2018), "Eleven states and the District of Columbia have sued the federal government over its proposed final rule to allow for association health plans that get around the Affordable Care Act's mandate to provide essential benefits." The original lawsuit was filed by the State of New York in the US District Court for the District of Columbia, with the US Department of Labor as the defendant. The States of Massachusetts, California, Delaware, Kentucky, Maryland,

New Jersey, Oregon, Pennsylvania, Virginia, and Washington, as well as the District of Columbia, all joined New York as plaintiffs in the case. The lawsuit, *New York v. U.S. Department of Labor*, challenged the status of an association of self-employed individuals as an employer and permitting employers in a geographic area who have no common business interest to collaborate to create AHPs.

In March 2019, the judge issued a ruling, finding in favor of the states' complaints. "In late March federal trial court judge John D. Bates of the District of Columbia agreed with the states . . . He set aside major provisions of the rule as inconsistent with federal law and unreasonable under the Administrative Procedure Act" (Keith 2019c, p. 894). The Trump administration appealed Judge Bates's ruling, but the restrictions he placed on AHPs will stay in place while the appeal is under consideration.

On November 19, 2019, a three-judge panel from the Court of Appeals for the District of Columbia heard oral arguments regarding the case. The plaintiffs contended that the federal Employee Retirement Income Security Act (ERISA) of 1974 set clear standards for employer-provided health insurance plans. According to the US Department of Labor (n.d.), "ERISA is a federal law that sets minimum standards for most voluntarily established retirement and health plans in private industry to provide protection for individuals in these plans."

Jost (2019) has reported that "under ERISA, an employee welfare benefit plan must generally be established and maintained by an employer for its employees." The ACA amended the law by differentiating between two types of employers: large employers, with more than 50 employees, and small employers, with between 2 and 50, and the rules governing health plans are different for them. "Historically, and under the Public Health Service Act, AHPs that covered individuals followed individual-market regulations and those that covered small groups followed small-group-market regulations." A central purpose of the changes made by the Trump administration was to allow AHPs to qualify as large employers, even though each of the employers within the association was either a small employer or a self-employed person. Jost continues, "It will likely be several months before the court decides the case."

Steps Individual States Have Taken to Buffer the Impacts of the Trump Administration's Changes

While the guidelines for STLD plans were established by the new rules issued by the Trump administration, individual states have the authority to further regulate these plans within their borders. Palanker, Kona, and Curran (2019) have analyzed the steps individual states have taken: "Twenty-two states limit the initial duration of a short-term plan to less than the federal limit of 12 months" (p. 2). Further, they found that Colorado and Connecticut require that these plans meet the standard of providing all essential health benefits established by the ACA. California has taken a more stringent approach: "But legislators in California concluded that the drawbacks of short-term plans outweigh any potential benefits, especially since consumers transitioning between coverage can buy ACA-compliant plans through special-enrollment periods. California banned short-term plans, so such plans may no longer be sold."

Eight other states and the District of Columbia limit these plans to a duration of six months or less. Five states and the District of Columbia prohibit the "stacking" of these plans, under which individuals purchase sequential short-term plans that in combination give substantially longer coverage. The main opposition to these changes was from insurance agents and brokers and the short-term plans themselves. Palanker, Kona, and Curran (2019, p. 7) conclude, "In states that take no steps to protect consumers, premium costs for ACA-compliant coverage are likely to rise and consumers will discover too late that their short-term plan does not provide the protection they expect . . . Although the effects of these state actions on the broader insurance markets is still unknown, these efforts show that regulating the short-term market is feasible."

California has gone beyond simply prohibiting short-term plans in resisting the Trump administration's changes. It has taken the major step of establishing a statewide individual mandate, requiring most residents either to have health insurance or to pay a tax penalty. "The new individual mandate for Californians starts in 2020. The penalty for not having insurance will mirror the one under the Affordable Care Act, which was $695 per adult (and $347.50 per child under 18) or 2.5% of annual household income, whichever is greater. That can amount to thousands of dollars a year" (Ostrov and Ibarra 2019).

California will use the funds received through the mandate penalty plus other state funds to provide "state-based tax credits for roughly 922,000 people who purchase insurance through Covered California." This funding will provide additional assistance to low-income households that already qualify for federal premium tax credits. In addition, "California will become the first state to offer financial aid to middle-income enrollees who make between 400% and 600% of the federal poverty level—many of whom have been struggling to pay their premiums" (Ostrov and Ibarra 2019).

Becker and Ponce (2019, p. 5) reported an additional change in California: "To stabilize the private purchase market, in 2017 the California legislature passed AB 156, which maintained the state's three-month open enrollment period. In addition, California continued full funding for the state's health insurance Navigator Program to help Californians enroll in health coverage, despite the elimination of federal matching funds for the program." California now provides state funding for navigator programs throughout the state to assist clients in enrolling in the most appropriate plan for them, including Medi-Cal for those who are eligible. It May 2019, the state announced it would provide $6.3 million to support navigator programs throughout the state (Covered California 2019).

Largely as a result of these extra steps California has taken, Ostrov and Ibarra (2019) have reported that, for coverage in 2020, "premiums on California's health insurance exchange will rise by an average of 0.8% next year, the lowest increase in the agency's history." A report by Dietz and colleagues (2019, pp. 7–8) concludes, "As a result of the state individual mandate penalty and state subsidies keeping more people in the individual market, we project that premiums in the individual market will be 8.5 percent lower in 2022 than they otherwise would have been due to a healthier risk mix in the individual market . . . These California policies are projected to result in 770,000 more Californians with health insurance coverage in 2022 than if these policies were not in place."

Based on the steps by multiple states to regulate short-term health plans and the steps taken by California to countermand many of the Trump administration's efforts to weaken the ACA, it appears that it is still possible to achieve market stability and enrollment sustenance. There are, however, two additional steps the Trump administration has taken in an attempt to weaken or even possibly to revoke the benefits created by the ACA. I will address these threats in the following chapter.

EIGHT

Two More Attempts to Defeat Key Elements of the Affordable Care Act

AS DESCRIBED in earlier chapters, Republicans in Congress, with both moral and administrative support from President Trump, made multiple, ultimately unsuccessful, attempts to repeal core aspects of the ACA. Instead, the Trump administration enacted several regulatory changes, such as association health plans and short-term health plans. Congress elected to block funding for reimbursing insurance companies for both the cost-sharing reductions mandated by the ACA and for the risk corridors programs. Congress also revoked the tax penalty that was the enforcement mechanism for the individual mandate created by the ACA.

None of these efforts had substantial, long-term negative impacts on ACA enrollment or premiums. After the initial instability in 2018 of the health exchange premiums for silver-level plans as a consequence of the decision not to fund the cost-sharing reductions, stability returned to the exchange market in 2019 and 2020. In the face of these failures to weaken and destabilize the ACA, the Trump administration and congressional Republicans focused their efforts on two alternative approaches: substantially reducing Medicaid enrollment among able-bodied adults and invalidating the entire ACA through federal courts.

Authorizing States to Impose Work Requirements
on Able-Bodied, Adult Medicaid Enrollees

When the ACA was originally passed in 2010, one of its major actions was to fundamentally alter the focus of the Medicaid program. Originally, Medicaid provided government-funded health insurance to three impoverished groups: the elderly, those with disabilities, and families with young children. Under the original law, poor, able-bodied, non-elderly adults who did not have children were excluded from the program.

Under the ACA, all states' Medicaid programs would automatically have been expanded to include all people with incomes below 138% of the federal poverty level. Many states objected and filed suit against the federal government to block this mandatory expansion of eligibility. The Supreme Court heard the case, *National Federation of Independent Business v. Sebelius*, in 2012. It ruled that the mandatory expansion of Medicaid by every state was not permitted under the Constitution. Threatening states with the loss of their preexisting Medicaid funding constituted an unreasonable penalty. Accordingly, each state could elect of its own accord whether to expand Medicaid or not. As of August 2020, 38 states and the District of Columbia had legally adopted Medicaid expansion (Kaiser Family Foundation 2020).

As I discussed in chapter 7, on January 20, 2017, the day of his inauguration, President Trump issued Executive Order 13765. That order instructed "the Secretary of Health and Human Services (Secretary) and the heads of all other executive departments and agencies (agencies) with authorities and responsibilities under the [Affordable Care] Act [to] exercise all authority and discretion available to them to waive, defer, grant exemptions from, or delay the implementation of any provision or requirement of the Act that would impose a fiscal burden on any State." The Medicaid expansion was one of the central provisions of the ACA President Trump and his supporters in Congress hoped to weaken.

In March 2017, following the guidance in that order, Thomas E. Price, the secretary of Health and Human Services, and Seema Verma, the administrator of the Centers for Medicare & Medicaid Services (CMS), issued guidance to all state governors of the types of changes they would like the states to enact (2017): "The expansion of Medicaid through the Affordable Care Act (ACA) to non-disabled, working-age adults without dependent children was a clear departure from the core, historical mission of the program." To address that departure, they wrote, "today, we commit to ushering in a new era for the federal and state Medicaid partnership where states have more freedom to design programs that meet the spectrum of diverse needs of their Medicaid population."

The letter then provided some specific examples of the changes Price and Verma (2017) would support: "The best way to improve the long-term health of low-income Americans is to empower them with skills and employment. It is our intent to use existing Section 1115 demonstration authority to review and approve meritorious innovations that build on the human dignity that comes with training, employment and independence." Section 1115 of the Social Security Act authorizes "any experimental, pilot, or demonstration project which, in the judgment of the Secretary, is likely to assist in promoting the objectives of title . . . XIX" (Social Security Administration n.d.).

On November 7, 2017, Verma gave a speech at the annual conference of the National Association of Medicaid Directors (2017). In that address, she described Medicaid as a program "that needs to be preserved and protected for those who truly need it." She went on to criticize the Medicaid expansion that was enacted under the ACA: "The ACA moved millions of working-age, non-disabled adults into a program that was created to care for seniors in need, pregnant mothers, children and people with disabilities . . . The thought that a program designed for our most vulnerable citizens should be used as a vehicle to serve working age, able-bodied adults does not make sense." One of the principal means Verma encouraged states to use was 1115 waivers to initiate requirements that able-bodied adults who were not part of "those who truly need it" either be employed or engage in comparable activities on a regular basis to maintain Medicaid eligibility.

As described by Rosenbaum (2017), "The revamping of federal Medicaid 1115 demonstration policy . . . has emerged as the centerpiece of the Administration's strategy to undo the ACA expansion and to otherwise move toward a fundamental lessening of the Medicaid program's size and scope, and a redefinition of its goals." This strategy applied both to states that had adopted the Medicaid expansion under ACA and those that had not. Verma indicated that CMS would give "fast track" review to state applications for Section 1115 waivers to initiate these types of work requirements. Rosenbaum reasoned, "Her remarks left no doubt that achieving multiple state Medicaid work demonstrations, in both expansion and non-expansion states, is the Administration's chief goal." On January 11, 2018, CMS sent a letter to all state Medicaid directors "announcing a new policy designed to assist states in their efforts to improve Medicaid enrollee health and well-being through incentivizing work and community engagement among non-elderly, non-pregnant adult Medicaid beneficiaries who are eligible for Medicaid on a basis other than disability" (Neal 2018).

On January 12, 2018, Paul Mango, the chief principal deputy administrator of CMS, issued a letter approving Kentucky's application for an 1115 waiver (Mango 2018a). On February 2, CMS also approved imposing work requirements under Indiana's 1115 waiver application (HHS Press Office 2018).

As described by Madubuonwu, Chen, and Sommers (2019), "The program, part of the state's 'Kentucky HEALTH' [Kentucky's Medicaid program] Medicaid waiver, would have required nonelderly, nonexempt adults to participate in community engagement for 80 hours a month." Community engagement included a range of possible activities, including employment, actively seeking work, volunteering in the community, or enrolling in school. Medicaid enrollees who were responsible for caring for family members were granted an exemption from the work requirements. Any adult who did not complete these 80 hours would lose their Medicaid coverage until they could document that they had met the requirements for a period of 30 days. The Kentucky plan also imposed a small monthly premium (4% of income) on enrollees.

Rosenbaum (2018), after evaluating the details of Kentucky's proposed work requirements, concluded that "what is so striking about the Kentucky experiment is the lengths to which the state and its federal partner have gone to come up with a strategy, under the guise of experimentation, for selectively culling the Medicaid population." In light of the potential impacts of the new requirements, scheduled to go into effect in July 2018, unsurprisingly, a lawsuit challenging the new requirements was filed shortly after the waiver was approved.

On January 24, 2018, a group of 15 Medicaid enrollees from Kentucky filed a lawsuit, *Stewart v. Azar*, in the US District Court for the District of Columbia, challenging the work requirements under the Kentucky waiver. "The plaintiffs argue that the Kentucky waiver puts them at risk of losing Medicaid by creating new eligibility criteria that they contend are beyond HHS's authority" (Musumeci 2018).

On June 29, 2018, the court issued its opinion, granting the plaintiff's motion and "vacat[ing] the Secretary's approval of Kentucky HEALTH" (*Stewart v. Azar* 2018). Kentucky then submitted an amended waiver request to CMS, again requesting authority to initiate work requirements for its Medicaid enrollees. On November 20, 2018, CMS approved the amended waiver request for Kentucky HEALTH (Mango 2018b). The plaintiffs in *Stewart v. Azar* again filed a suit to block the revised waiver. On March 27, 2019, the court issued its ruling, again overturning CMS's approval of Kentucky's waiver request (Galewitz 2019a).

By November 2018, CMS had granted 1115 waivers for four states to impose work requirements on Medicaid enrollees: Arkansas, Indiana, Kentucky, and New Hampshire (Goldman et al. 2018). Seven other states had submitted applications for waiver requests that were under review by CMS. By November 2019, CMS had approved waiver applications from Michigan, Ohio, Utah, and Wisconsin. Eight additional states at this point had submitted waiver requests that were under review (Kaiser Family Foundation 2019).

Silvestri, Holland, and Ross (2018) analyzed the characteristics of the Medicaid population in the states that had requested work requirement waivers. They concluded that "almost all Medicaid-eligible individuals may already meet proposed work requirements or exemptions prior to implementation" (p. 1553). The percentage of Medicaid enrollees who were subject to the requirements ranged from 21.8% in Mississippi to

54% in New Hampshire. A substantial majority of these adults were already employed and were thus meeting the work requirements. Of these adults who were subject to the requirements, the percentage who were not already meeting the requirement ranged from a low of 1.6% in Arkansas to 10.6% in New Hampshire.

Chokshi and Katz (2018) responded to these analyses by comparing the proposed work requirements to the English Poor Laws of the sixteenth century.

> In 1563, Elizabethan English law distinguished between the deserving poor, or those who wanted to work but could not because of infirmity or lack of available work, and the idle poor, or those who were judged able to work but would not. While the deserving poor were to be aided, the idle poor were to be punished. Four hundred fifty years later, the United States is still debating which of the poor are deserving and what they are deserving of. One of the current battlegrounds is work requirements for Medicaid recipients to receive health insurance benefits.

An example of a state in which this characterization applies is Alabama. Alabama is one of the states that elected not to expand its Medicaid program under the ACA. Accordingly, the new work requirements Alabama proposed would affect extremely poor parents. Elderly and disabled adult enrollees would be exempt.

The Georgetown University Center for Children and Families (2018) analyzed the proposed work requirements in Alabama, with some very interesting findings: "Alabama is seeking federal permission through a Section 1115 Medicaid demonstration waiver to require parents and caregivers who rely on Medicaid to work 20 to 35 hours a week, prove they are looking or training for a job or do community service before receiving Medicaid." The analysis underscores the finding that Alabama has one of the most restrictive eligibility levels for these parents under traditional Medicaid. To qualify, a parent or family may earn no more than $3,740 per year, or about $312 per month.

Assuming that any parent who finds employment will earn the federal minimum wage of $7.25 per hour, if that parent works 20 hours per week, they would earn more than $600 per month. As described in the Georgetown analysis, "The proposal creates a Catch-22: Any parent working the 20 to 35 hours required would make too much money to qualify for Medicaid—but likely not enough to afford private insurance. The state estimates that just under 15,000 parents would be removed from Medicaid by the fifth year of the proposal. This number is likely too low" (2018). If the goal of Alabama's proposed waiver is simply to disqualify parents currently eligible for Medicaid, I can only concur with the analysis by Chokshi and Katz that the proposal reenacts the English Poor Laws. As of November 2019, Alabama's waiver is still under review at CMS.

As stringent as Alabama's proposed waiver is, Alker (2019a) has reported that Florida is considering even more stringent regulations. "A Florida House Committee recently (3/13) approved HB 955, on a party line vote, a bill that would authorize the Governor to seek a Section 1115 Medicaid waiver to impose likely the most punitive work reporting requirements in the nation on very poor parents receiving their health coverage through Medicaid." Under the bill proposed by the committee, the only parents currently covered under Medicaid who would be exempt from new work requirements would be those with a newborn child under 3 months of age. The bill would impose a requirement of a minimum of 20 hours per week on other parents. With Florida's minimum wage set at $8.46 per hour, a parent working the minimum of 20 hours per week would earn about $677 per month. As in Alabama, this income would be greater than the maximum allowed for Medicaid eligibility, leading the parent to lose Medicaid coverage.

On May 1, 2019, Alker (2019b) reported that the proposed legislation had passed the Florida House by a largely party-line vote of 71-44. However, the Florida Senate did not take up the proposed legislation before adjourning, so Florida did not submit its waiver request to CMS.

The first state that actually imposed Medicaid work requirements after receiving an 1115 waiver from CMS was Arkansas. Arkansas has taken a somewhat different approach to Medicaid than most other states. Arkansas elected to expand Medicaid under the ACA to all individuals with incomes less than 138% of FPL. To do this, in 2013 Arkansas was granted a separate 1115 waiver under which it would enroll all eligible non-disabled adults under age 65 in a private health insurance plan, Arkansas Works (Centers for Medicare & Medicaid Services n.d.). Those with incomes between 100% and 138% of FPL would have to pay a monthly premium that was no more than 2% of household income.

In April 2018, Arkansas was granted a second 1115 waiver, authorizing the state to initiate a work requirement. "The new requirements were phased in for most enrollees ages 30–49 beginning in June 2018 and for individuals ages 19–29 starting in January 2019. Unless exempt, enrollees must engage in 80 hours of work or other qualifying activities each month and must report their work or exemption status by the 5th of the following month using an online portal; as of mid-December 2018, they also may report by phone" (Rudowitz, Musumeci, and Hall 2019). A core aspect of the Arkansas requirement is the two-phase requirement: the enrollee must first complete the work requirement, and then must report compliance with the requirement. Failure to meet either requirement would lead to loss of Medicaid coverage.

Between June and December 2018, 18,164 Medicaid enrollees in Arkansas lost their coverage because they failed to report their work hours, even though most of them had been employed the minimum 20 hours per week or more. Those who lost coverage in 2018 were eligible to reapply for coverage in 2019; however, only 1,910 of them had regained their coverage. By February 2019, when the age range of those required to meet the work requirements was fully expanded, 116,229 adults were subject to the work requirements. This number comprised nearly half of the 238,870 adults covered under Arkansas Works. Those enrolled in Arkansas Works who were 50 years or older were not subject to the work requirements (Rudowitz, Musumeci, and Hall 2019).

Data from February 2019 cited by Rudowitz, Musumeci, and Hall (2019) showed that nearly 90% of those who first became subject to the requirements in 2019 failed to report the required 80 hours of work for the month. Nearly all of these individuals had failed to register any work hours, either online or by phone. Sommers and colleagues (2019) conducted a telephone survey of nearly 6,000 low-income adults, approximately half of whom were from Arkansas. Among Arkansas residents age 30–49 years, 32.9% reported not having heard anything about the new work requirements. Even fewer of the respondents aged 19–29 years had heard of them. Among those who had, about half were unsure whether the requirements applied to them. Among those who had received word from the state that they were required to report work or other qualifying activities, only half were actually doing so.

As compared to low-income adults in comparison states, the rate of employment among those in Arkansas had not changed during the period the work requirements were in effect. It appears the purported goal of increasing employment among low-income adults was not attained. Sommers and colleagues (2019, p. 1080) identified the predominant cause of the failure to report work hours among those in Arkansas: "Our descriptive results indicate that the implementation of this policy was plagued by confusion among many enrollees, a finding consistent with qualitative research. Lack of Internet access was also a barrier to reporting information to the state." They also reported that "one third of persons who were subject to the policy had not heard anything about it, and 44% of the target population was unsure whether the requirements applied to them."

The Arkansas work requirements came to an end in March 2019. When Judge James Boasberg issued his second ruling blocking Kentucky from implementing Medicaid work requirements, he also ruled in a second lawsuit, *Gresham v. Azar*, that challenged the imposition of work requirements in Arkansas (Galewitz 2019a). The judge "found that the Secretary's approval of the Arkansas demonstration (Arkansas Works), and the Secretary's reapproval of the Kentucky demonstration (Kentucky HEALTH), was in each case arbitrary and capricious, and he vacated and remanded both demonstrations back to the Secretary" (Schneider 2019). Effective April 1, 2019, no Medicaid enrollee in Arkansas could be disenrolled for failure to meet the work requirements, and those who had previously been disenrolled had their coverage restored.

This was not the last time a judge would block a state's implementation of Medicaid work requirements. "On July 29th—for the fourth time—Judge James Boasberg of the United States District Court for the District of Columbia, in Philbrick v Azar, vacated HHS approval of an

1115 Medicaid work experiment waiver. This time it was New Hampshire's approval that fell" (Rosenbaum 2019). Rosenbaum goes on to describe Judge Boasberg's growing frustration with these lawsuits. "Judge Boasberg's decision had more than a hint of weariness to it; as he noted 'the issues presented in this case are all too familiar' . . . Indeed, Judge Boasberg noted, the Secretary's failure was even more glaring in New Hampshire, whose work requirements are 'more exacting than Kentucky's and Arkansas's.'"

Despite these rulings, as of November 2019, Arizona, Indiana, Michigan, Ohio, Utah, and Wisconsin received approval of their 1115 waiver proposals to implement Medicaid work requirements. An additional eight states had waiver applications pending at CMS. Support for granting these waivers apparently had not weakened within CMS. "Seema Verma, the Trump administration's top Medicaid official, Tuesday sharply attacked critics of her plan to force some Medicaid enrollees to work, a policy that led to thousands of people losing coverage in Arkansas. 'We cannot allow those who prefer the status quo to weaponize the legal system against state innovation,' the administrator of the Centers for Medicare & Medicaid Services said in a fiery speech to the nation's 56 state and territorial Medicaid directors in Washington, D.C." (Galewitz 2019b).

Verma goes on to voice her criticism of those opposing the imposition of Medicaid work requirements in very sharp terms: "Part of my mission is to fight such underhanded tactics and preserve the right of states to shape your programs in ways that are consistent with the needs of your residents, your cultures and your values. Anything less stifles innovation" (Galewitz 2019b). Seema Verma, as the senior administrator in the Centers for Medicare and Medicaid Services, is following the vituperative approach President Trump and many congressional Republicans have taken in response to the Medicaid expansion and other central components of the ACA.

Verma's passionate advocacy for imposing work requirements was reflected in her decision announced on December 12, 2019, to grant South Carolina a waiver to combine a partial expansion of Medicaid financial eligibility with the imposition of work requirements on all parents with children. As recounted in the *New York Times* by Goodnough (2019a), "Ms. Verma traveled to Greenville, S.C., on Thursday to announce the decision with Gov. Henry McMaster, a Republican. In a statement, she predicted that the work requirements 'will lift South Carolinians out of poverty by encouraging as many as possible to participate in the booming Trump economy.'" Governor McMaster echoed Verma's comments: "In this economy, there is no excuse for the able-bodied not to be working."

As reported by Alker (2019c), "The families who will be disproportionately harmed are more likely to be households headed by women, African American, and living in rural areas." The South Carolina waiver did expand Medicaid eligibility to all parents with incomes below the FPL, so long as they meet the work requirement. Notably, the waiver granted to South Carolina also expanded Medicaid eligibility to approximately 14,000 adults who are chronically homeless, many of whom suffer from mental illness or substance abuse. These homeless adults would also have to meet the work requirement, either by working or performing other qualifying activities, to be eligible. Even with this additional eligibility expansion, it is likely the same court constraints will be applied to South Carolina as have been applied to the other states.

As reported by Goodnough (2020), "A federal appeals court panel on Friday [February 14] unanimously upheld a lower court's ruling striking down work rules for Medicaid recipients in Arkansas . . . A three-judge panel of the United States Court of Appeals for the District of Columbia Circuit found that approval of the Arkansas work requirement by the health and human services secretary, Alex M. Azar, was 'arbitrary and capricious' because it did not address how the program would promote the objective of Medicaid as defined under federal law: providing health coverage to the poor." While the case applied only to the work requirements imposed in Arkansas, it had major implications for other states with either approved or pending waivers. "While litigation has not been filed with respect to these waivers yet, it is very important to be aware that all of these cases would be filed here in DC and be assigned to Judge Boasberg," the district court judge who initially struck down the Arkansas work requirements and also issued rulings striking down work requirements in New Hampshire and Kentucky (Alker 2020).

A Final Effort to Repeal the ACA—the Case of *Texas v. United States*

After final passage of the ACA in 2010, groups opposed to the act were quick to challenge its legality on constitutional grounds, primarily focusing on the requirement that each state expand its Medicaid program to include all adults with incomes less than 138% of the FPL. The second challenge was to the constitutionality of the individual mandate. The lawsuits challenging these aspects of the ACA were combined into one case: *National Federation of Independent Business v. Sebelius*.

After working its way through federal district courts and appeals courts, the case was heard and decided by the Supreme Court. The issue at stake in the question of the individual mandate was this: "The plaintiffs argued that individual choices in matters of health insurance were not part of interstate commerce and therefore were not covered under Article 1 Section 8 of the US Constitution, which grants the federal government authority 'to regulate commerce . . . among the several states.'" The court issued its decision in June 2012:

> The Court agreed that the interstate commerce clause of Article 1, Section 8, did not apply to the decision to purchase health insurance, as individual decisions of this type are not part of interstate commerce. However, while the federal government may not force someone to acquire health insurance, it can levy an extra tax on those who elect not to obtain coverage. Even though ACA legislation identified the required payment as a "penalty," it was included under the federal government's authority under Article 1, Section 8, to "lay and collect taxes." (Barr 2016, p. 14)

Requiring someone to have health insurance is not allowed under the Constitution. Assessing a tax penalty for not having insurance is allowed. One part of the individual mandate as contained in the ACA was unconstitutional; one part, the tax penalty, was not.

What, though, if the tax penalty were revoked via legislation while the mandate to have health insurance remained? That would appear to leave the ACA with one component that was not permitted under the Constitution. Would the inclusion of a component that violated the Constitution mean that the entire ACA legislation is unconstitutional? This is precisely the question that plaintiffs raised in a lawsuit filed in February 2018.

In December 2017, the Republican Congress passed and President Trump signed the Tax Cuts and Jobs Act of 2017. One component of the act was to remove the tax penalty for not carrying health insurance, effective January 1, 2019. With the tax penalty removed, the individual mandate to have health insurance remained. On February 26, 2018, Texas and 19 other states filed a lawsuit in the United States District Court for the North District of Texas, *Texas v. United States*. The plaintiffs argued that, because the individual mandate remained in the ACA while the tax penalty had been removed and since the Supreme Court had ruled that the individual mandate was unconstitutional, the continued presence of a section of the ACA that violates the Constitution means that the entire ACA violates the Constitution.

In addition to the 20 states acting as plaintiffs in the case, two individuals also joined the suit. Each lives in Texas and had purchased health insurance through the ACA exchange, not qualifying for PTC subsidies. These individuals asserted that they felt an obligation under the law to purchase ACA-compliant health insurance, even after the tax penalty had been revoked. They would have preferred the opportunity to purchase private health insurance in the open market without restrictions included in the ACA. Accordingly, they asked the judge to declare the entire ACA as unconstitutional, based on its inclusion of the unconstitutional individual mandate.

This challenge to the ACA raises the legal issue of "severability." Before the Supreme Court had issued its opinion in the lawsuit challenging the constitutionality of the individual mandate, Gluck and Graetz (2012) published an Op-Ed in the *New York Times* titled "The Severability Doctrine." In it they addressed the issue of severability if one part of a law is found to be unconstitutional. "The Supreme Court has long affirmed a 'presumption in favor of severability,' meaning that when it rules that a statutory provision is unconstitutional, the decision should affect as little of the law as possible." The court's decision in *National Federation of Independent Business v. Sebelius* appears to be consistent with this principle. The court ruled that the constitutional violation of the individual mandate did not invalidate the remainder of the ACA legislation.

In *Texas v. United States*, the plaintiffs argued just the opposite. With the tax penalty removed, the fact that the text of the individual mandate remained in the law and had been ruled unconstitutional, therefore rendered the entire law was unconstitutional. They asserted that the individual mandate was inseverable from the remainder of the law. The plaintiffs asked the court to rule that the entire ACA was unconstitutional based on this principle.

In May 2018, before hearing oral arguments in the case, the court allowed 16 states, led by California, as well as the District of Columbia to intervene in the case to defend the constitutionality of the ACA. These states argued that they would lose billions of dollars in federal funds under the ACA if the law were invalidated.

The intervention of these states as defendants proved to be timely. In the summer of 2018, before Judge Reed O'Connor heard oral arguments, the Trump administration added another twist to the case. "In June the Department of Justice had, in a surprise move, agreed with the plaintiffs that the mandate is unconstitutional but argued that only the ACA's guaranteed issue and community rating provisions, as well as its ban on preexisting condition exclusion clauses, must be invalidated" (Jost 2018). Instead of defending the constitutionality of the ACA, the Trump administration was arguing in favor of the plaintiffs in the case.

On September 5, Judge O'Connor heard oral arguments in the case. On December 14, he issued his ruling. As reported by de Vogue and Luhby (2018), "A federal judge in Texas said on Friday that the Affordable Care Act's individual coverage mandate is unconstitutional and that the rest of the law therefore cannot stand." The authors went on to report, "Legal experts say the ruling won't immediately affect Americans' health coverage, and a group of states led by California is already vowing to appeal."

That evening, President Trump posted on his Twitter account (Trump 2018) "As I predicted all along, Obamacare has been struck down as an UNCONSTITUTIONAL disaster! Now Congress must pass a STRONG law that provides GREAT healthcare and protects pre-existing conditions. Mitch and Nancy, get it done!"

On December 30, "The federal judge who declared the Affordable Care Act's individual coverage mandate unconstitutional earlier this month issued an order on Sunday saying despite his previous ruling the law can remain in effect pending appeal" (Sullivan and Luhby 2018). California attorney general Xavier Becerra responded by saying that California and the other defending states would file their appeal "expeditiously."

In April 2019, Drew Altman and Mollyann Brodie of the Kaiser Family Foundation reported the results of a national poll on the public's support for the ACA (2019). Among Republicans, 7 respondents out of 10 reported that they wanted Congress to repeal the ACA and for the Supreme Court to declare the ACA unconstitutional. However, the authors also reported that "majorities of Republicans like many elements of the ACA—especially closing the 'doughnut hole' in Medicare prescription drug coverage (80%), eliminating copayments for preventive services (68%), and keeping young adults under 26 on their parents' plans (66%) and subsidies for low- and middle-income households (63%)." They also found near-majority support for keeping the protections for preexisting conditions, even if the Supreme Court were to find the ACA unconstitutional based on the individual mandate.

California and the other original defendants, joined by four additional states, appealed the case to the Fifth Circuit Court of Appeals in New Orleans. Given the results of the November 2018 elections and the election of a Democratic majority in the House, the court also allowed the House of Representatives to join the 20 states and the District of Columbia in defense of the ACA. Twenty organizations, including the American Hospital Association, the American Medical Association, the

American Cancer Society, the American Association of Retired Persons, and several insurance companies submitted amicus briefs on behalf of the defendants.

While the plaintiffs and the defendants were preparing for the appeals court hearing, the Department of Justice made an unexpected change in its position regarding the lawsuit. Recall from above that "the Department of Justice had, in a surprise move, agreed with the plaintiffs that the mandate is unconstitutional but argued that only the ACA's guaranteed issue and community rating provisions, as well as its ban on preexisting condition exclusion clauses, must be invalidated" (Jost 2018). "In yet another unexpected twist in litigation over the constitutionality of the Affordable Care Act (ACA), the Department of Justice (DOJ) took the new and stunning position that the entire ACA should be invalidated because the individual mandate penalty has been set to $0 . . . The DOJ now fully agrees that a December 2018 decision—where a district court declared the entire ACA to be invalid—should be affirmed and upheld by the Fifth Circuit" (Keith 2019a). It was not clear at the time why the DOJ had changed its position regarding how much of the ACA should be invalidated based on the circuit court's ruling.

The inconsistency in the DOJ's approach to the appeal of the circuit court's ruling was to show itself again. At the time the court of appeals conducted its hearing in July, "the DOJ, by taking yet another new legal position in the lawsuit, injected a significant degree of additional uncertainty and confusion into the proceedings. The district court's ruling was universally viewed as applying nationwide (rather than only the plaintiff states and individuals). But last week, the DOJ indicated its new view that Judge O'Connor's decision applied only to the 18 plaintiff states and two individuals" (Keith 2019b). It was unclear how the DOJ had determined that the unconstitutionality of the individual mandate would invalidate the entire ACA but only in those states who had joined the lawsuit as plaintiffs.

On July 9, 2019, the three-judge panel of the court of appeals heard oral arguments from both the plaintiffs and the defendants on Texas v. United States. The oral arguments centered on three basic questions (Keith 2019b):

1. Do all the parties have legal standing to bring or defend the lawsuit?

To be granted standing, a party must have sustained an injury because of the law. The circuit court judge had ruled only that the two individual plaintiffs from Texas had legal standing to bring the suit. He had not ruled on whether Texas and the other states acting as plaintiffs had legal standing to bring the suit. Likewise, the judge had not ruled as to whether the states defending the suit had legal standing. Since the House of Representatives had entered the suit after the judge had issued his ruling, the plaintiffs questioned whether the House had legal standing to participate.

2. Does the revocation of the individual mandate tax penalty make the individual mandate that remained part of the ACA unconstitutional?

This is the central question of the lawsuit and is based largely on the Supreme Court's 2012 ruling in *National Federation of Independent Business v. Sebelius*.

3. If the individual mandate is unconstitutional, is it severable from the remainder of the ACA, or does it make the entire ACA unconstitutional?

The issue of severability is central to the case. "Supreme Court precedent on severability directs courts to limit damage to a statute and be guided by congressional intent" (Keith 2019b). This principle was addressed in further detail by an amici curiae brief filed in June 2018 (Adler et al. 2018): "The cornerstone of severability doctrine is congressional intent. Under current Supreme Court doctrine, a court must offer its best guess on what Congress would have wanted for the rest of the statute if a single provision is rendered unenforceable." The authors go on to argue, "An unbroken line of Supreme Court severability precedent rests on two foundational principles. First, courts must 'try not to nullify more of a legislature's work than is necessary' because '[a] ruling of unconstitutionality frustrates the intent of the elected representatives of the people.' . . . Second, 'the touchstone for any decision about remedy is legislative intent', for a court cannot 'use its remedial powers to circumvent the intent of the legislature.'"

In their analysis of *Texas v. United States*, a group of senior legal scholars working with the Constitutional Accountability Center, "a think tank, law firm, and action center dedicated to fulfilling the progressive promise of our Constitution's text and history," argue that some clearly established legal precedents apply to the case (Wydra et al. 2019). "In striking down the entire Affordable Care Act, the district court disregarded the clearly expressed intent of the democratically elected representatives of the People . . . Even if the Court concludes that the mandate is unconstitutional, it should look to Congress's intent to determine the appropriate remedy. Congress's intent here could not be clearer: the rest of the law should stand in the absence of an enforceable mandate."

Abby Goodnough (2019b) reported in the *New York Times* on the oral arguments presented in the hearing before the Court of Appeals. "A panel of federal appeals court judges on Tuesday sounded likely to uphold a lower-court ruling that a central provision of the Affordable Care Act—the requirement that most people have health insurance—is unconstitutional. But it was harder to discern how the court might come down on a much bigger question: whether the rest of the sprawling health law must fall if the insurance mandate does."

Nicole Huberfeld (2019), professor of health law, ethics, and human rights at the School of Public Health and professor of law at the School of Law at Boston University, has analyzed the issue of severability. She refers to the Supreme Court's decision in the case of *National Federation of Independent Business v. Sebelius*, in which the court ruled that the ACA's mandate that all states expand their Medicaid program to include all adults with incomes under 138% of FPL was a violation of the constitution. She argues that "the Court held that mandatory expansion of Medicaid eligibility unconstitutionally 'coerced' states, ruling instead that states should be allowed to opt in or out. The Medicaid aspect of the NFIB ruling indicates that the ACA is 'severable'—even if parts are eliminated, the remainder of the law would continue to operate." If the Supreme Court had adopted the approach of inseverability in its ruling in *National Federation of Independent Business v. Sebelius*, it would have invalidated the entire ACA in 2012. It did not do so. As Huberfeld argued, if the Medicaid violation was severable, then it is only reasonable to assume that the individual mandate is as well.

The court of appeals issued its ruling on December 18, 2019 (*Texas v. United States* 2019). The ruling was joined by two of the three justices, with one justice dissenting. The court ruled that both the plaintiffs and the defendants have standing in the case. The ruling then states, "The individual mandate is unconstitutional because it can no longer be read as a tax, and there is no other constitutional provision that justifies this exercise of congressional power." The ruling continued, "On the severability question, we remand to the district court to provide additional analysis of the provisions of the ACA as they currently exist." The court then stated that it was "directing the district court to employ a finer toothed comb on remand and conduct a more searching inquiry into which provisions of the ACA Congress intended to be inseverable from the individual mandate." It thus would have been up to Judge O'Connor, the judge in Texas who issued the initial ruling, to go through the ACA legislation in detail and to indicate which parts are severable from the mandate ruling and which are inseverable. The dissenting justice argued that the entirety of the ACA was clearly severable from the mandate and that remanding the case for further analysis "will unnecessarily prolong this litigation and the concomitant uncertainty over the future of the healthcare sector."

It perhaps was not surprising that the appeals court upheld the district court's decision that, absent the mandate tax penalty, the mandate itself is unconstitutional. It was somewhat more surprising that the court declined to rule on the severability issue. In reporting the decision, Rovner (2019) referred to a quote from Senator Lamar Alexander, a Republican from Tennessee: "I am not aware of a single senator who said they were voting to repeal Obamacare when they voted to eliminate the individual mandate penalty." Alexander thus confirmed that it was not the intent of Congress to repeal or weaken the ACA when it repealed the individual mandate tax penalty.

In January, the Democratic states along with the House of Representatives that had taken the case to the appeals court then appealed that court's decision to the Supreme Court. "The appeal asks the court to review the case quickly—during the court's current session—a schedule that would allow the outcome to be final before the 2020 presidential election" (Sanger-Katz 2020). California attorney general Xavier Becerra is leading the effort. On January 21, the Supreme Court turned down the request for rapid review (Liptak 2020). As reported by Liptak and Goodnough on March 3, 2020, "The Supreme Court agreed on Monday to hear a third major challenge to the Affordable Care Act, setting up likely arguments this fall in a case that could wipe out President Barack Obama's signature domestic achievement . . . The Supreme Court did not say when it would hear the case, but under its ordinary practices, arguments would be held in the fall and a decision would land in the spring or summer of 2021."

The Supreme Court heard oral arguments in the case on November 10, 2020. Coming a week after the election of Joseph Biden Jr. as the next president, the Court's hearing gained wide attention. As described by Keith (2020), the questions posed by the Justices addressed the same three questions identified above by Keith in her report of the Appeals Court consideration of the case: whether the parties to the suit have legal standing; whether the revocation of the individual mandate tax penalty makes the individual mandate unconstitutional; and, if so, whether the mandate is severable from the remainder of the ACA.

Of these, perhaps the most salient point is the severability of the mandate should the Court find it unconstitutional. Writing in the *New York Times*, Liptak (2020) reported the Court's questioning during oral arguments: "Both Chief Justice John G. Roberts Jr. and Justice Brett M. Kavanaugh said striking down the so-called individual mandate did not require the rest of the law to be struck down as well. 'Congress left the rest of the law intact when it lowered the penalty to zero,' Chief Justice Roberts said. Justice Kavanaugh made a similar point. 'It does seem fairly clear that the proper remedy would be to sever the mandate provision and leave the rest of the act in place.'"

Jost (2020) came to a similar conclusion: "It was here that the Court tipped its hand most clearly. Both Chief Justice Roberts and Justice Kavanaugh suggested that they believed the remainder of the ACA was severable from the mandate." The Court is expected to deliver its ruling some time in spring or early summer of 2021.

With Joe Biden elected as president in the November elections and with Democrats maintaining a reduced but persistent majority in the House, the possibility of amending the ACA to address the issue of the mandate will largely depend on the Senate. Even if the Republicans were to maintain a slim majority in the Senate, President Biden has committed to reestablishing the type of bipartisan cooperation he experienced personally during his six terms as senator from Delaware. As reported in the *New York Times* by Herndon (2020), Biden has "cast the moment as a chance for the country to excise the political division Mr. Trump has stoked, promising to repair the ideological, racial, and geographic fissures that have grown into chasms since 2016."

If Congress were to impose a small penalty for failing to maintain health insurance (as compared to the penalty of $695 or 2.5% of income, whichever is greater, as under the original law), the issue of the constitutionality of the individual mandate would become moot. Alternatively, Congress and the president could agree to remove the individual mandate from the ACA. Removal of the mandate would likely have little impact on continued enrollment in health insurance under the ACA. As described by Keith (2020), "While Congress thought the individual mandate was crucial in adopting the ACA in 2010, it turns out that the ACA subsidies can work without the mandate. This was confirmed by the [Congressional Budget Office] estimates in 2017 . . . ." We will simply need to wait to see the course history takes.

NINE

Bridging the Health Care Chasm

IN THE introduction, I referenced a quotation from Jonathan Oberlander (2019): "Intensifying partisan polarization in Congress has made it more difficult to forge compromise, leading to more legislative deadlock . . . The ideological chasm between Democrats and Republicans in Congress makes it difficult to find common ground on policy."

From my perspective, the issues I addressed in the previous few chapters—the defunding of cost-sharing reductions, imposing Medicaid work requirements, and the repeal of the individual mandate penalty and the lawsuit in Texas to invalidate the entire Affordable Care Act—have provided clear confirmation of Oberlander's conclusion. As of the 2020 elections, the two parties in Congress were standing on opposite sides of an ever-widening political and cultural chasm.

I represent that chasm metaphorically with an image of the chasm created by the Rio Grande as it courses through Los Alamos Canyon near the San Ildefonso Pueblo in northern New Mexico. Imagine two congressional leaders—one Republican and one Democrat—standing on opposite sides of the plateau that overlooks the canyon. They are far enough apart that it would be difficult for either to see the other, let alone speak with the other. To me, that image represents the situation in

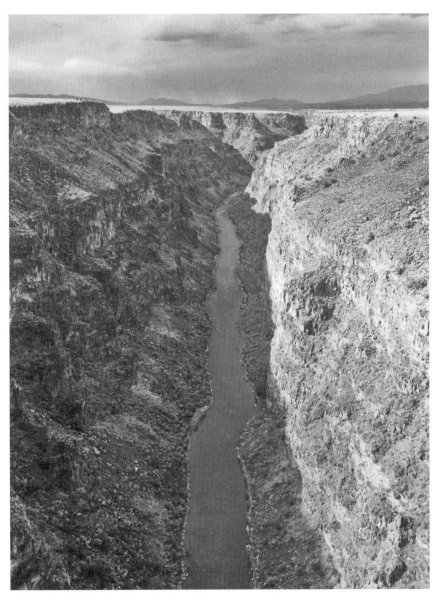
Los Alamos Canyon. Photo by Donald A Barr

which our country found itself with respect to the ACA and national health care policy.

Now imagine that, following the election of Joseph Biden as president, each leader decided, of their own accord, to walk upstream, to where the canyon narrows. At that point, the sides of the chasm are considerably closer to each other. Each could see the other clearly and speak with the other without having to yell or shout. What might they talk about?

What if each, of their own accord, suggested building a bridge across the chasm so they could meet to discuss possible areas of agreement? How might they approach such a task? What type of bridge might they build? Who would do the work?

To explore possible answers to these questions, again metaphorically, I thumbed through a book by Judith Dupré titled *Bridges: A History of the World's Most Spectacular Spans* (2017). I looked at images of ancient Roman bridges, more modern ones such as the Brooklyn Bridge and the Golden Gate Bridge, and the incredibly long bridges in China and Japan.

Then someone told me about the Q'eswachaka Rope Bridge, which spans the Apurimac Canyon in Peru. "Q'eswachaka or Keshwa Chaca, this is one of the only remaining examples of the Incan hand-woven bridges once common in the Incan road system. Made of woven grass, the bridge spans 118 feet and hangs 60 feet above the canyon's rushing river" (Atlas Obscura website 2020) and is pictured below.

The bridge is constructed of a series of ropes made from hay harvested locally. As the ropes weaken over time with exposure to the weather, each year the villagers come together to construct a new bridge, as seen in a YouTube video posted by Great Big Story (2017). It is the job of families on both sides of the canyon to harvest hay, cure it, and then fashion it into a series of long, thin ropes. On a given morning each year, all the thin ropes are brought together and woven into six thick ones—four to function as the footbridge and two as handrails.

The key to building this bridge is that villagers on either side of the canyon agree to cooperate on its construction. The first step is to carry a thin rope from one side of the canyon to the other. Villagers on one

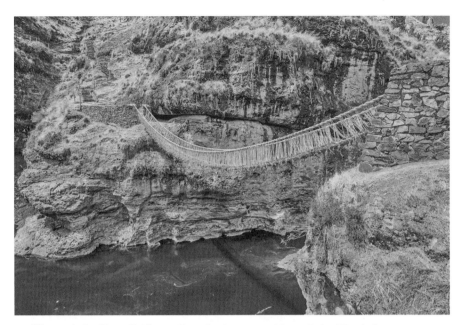
Q'eswachaka Rope Bridge. Wikimedia Commons; ©Joerg Steber/iStockphoto

side attach this rope to a thick rope, and villagers on the other side then use the thin rope to pull the thick one across the canyon. This process is repeated until all six thick ropes span the canyon.

The next step is for one villager from each side of the canyon to sit on the four thick ropes and weave them together with short, thin ropes. A villager in the video describes this process (Great Big Story 2017): "We work to inch our way towards the middle where both ends meet." Once the two weavers meet in the middle, the bridge is nearly done. Thin ropes are then used to make a safety mesh between the handrails and the footbridge. When the process is complete, the villager describes what comes next: "We always celebrate our new bridge by singing and dancing. I love the bridge, and right now I'm proud and happy that it's being renewed. This bridge makes us all proud. Long live the bridge. May it last forever." This process has been going on for generations, and it looks like it will continue to do so for generations yet to come. Can congressional leaders learn anything from the Peruvian villagers' art of collaborative bridge making?

If I were to apply the metaphor of the rope bridge to the challenge of addressing the current health care divide, I would suggest that congressional leaders could take the following steps:

1. Each side would agree to begin working on changes in health policy that they could support (i.e., curing hay to make the thin rope).
2. The two sides would work together to weave these potential changes into four potential modifications of current policy that each side could agree to (i.e., weave the thick ropes).
3. The two sides would agree to collaborate in building momentum for these changes, without altering the current system in a major way (i.e., collaboratively stretch the thick ropes across the canyon and weave them together to make a footbridge).
4. Once the initial policy changes were agreed to, each side would agree to participate in an ongoing forum in both the Senate and in the House to explore and discuss health care issues on which there might be bipartisan consensus (i.e., add the handrails and safety mesh siding to prevent falls).

There is consistent data nationally to suggest that some health policy issues have relatively wide, bipartisan support. In the introduction I cited work by Blendon, Benson, and McMurtry (2019) documenting that the biggest health care issue for the American public is cost, with more than two-thirds of respondents indicating that reducing health care costs should be a top national priority. There is not strong bipartisan agreement on how to do so, but there is an impetus for finding a way to reduce health care costs. I suggest that there are specific policy issues involving health care costs that could provide the "ropes" by which a bridge across the chasm might be constructed. Below I identify and discuss potential policy steps to address these issues.

Fixing the Family Glitch

Under the ACA, most employees continue to obtain their health insurance as a fringe benefit through their employers. Those who do not have employer-provided coverage available to them are then eligible to go onto the health exchanges established by ACA, either state based or federal. Those individuals and families who acquire coverage through an exchange and who have household incomes between 100% and 400% of the federal poverty level are then eligible for a federal premium tax credit (PTC) subsidy.

Under ACA, for those who have employer-provided health insurance available to them that is "affordable," neither they nor their family members are eligible to obtain coverage through the exchanges. The ACA defines "affordable" as no more than 9.78% of yearly income to cover the employee's share of the annual health insurance premium. If the employer offers insurance that costs more than 9.78% and is therefore not "affordable," these employees are eligible to go to the exchange and acquire coverage with any PTCs they may be eligible for.

There is a glitch in how this works. The definition of "affordable" applies only to the premium employees pay for individual coverage. If the share of the premium for individual coverage is less than 9.78% of their income but the premium to cover their entire family is greater than 9.78%, they still meet the definition of having access to "affordable" insurance, and neither they nor their family are eligible for coverage through the exchanges, with or without PTCs.

As an example, let us consider a family of four with Mr. A, age 48, employed and making $50,000 per year, Mrs. A, age 46, at home without employment, and two children, aged 15 and 12. Based on the national income distribution for 2018, the A household is making approximately 81% of the national median household income (Guzman 2019). According to data compiled by the Kaiser Family Foundation (2019), in 2019 the average employee contribution nationally for individual coverage obtained from an employer was $1,242. Assuming Mr. A paid the average premium, single coverage through his employer would cost him 2.5% of his annual income, which makes it "affordable" under ACA standards. If Mr. A elected to cover his entire family through his employer, the average employee share of the family premium would be $6,015, 12% of his annual income.

In addition to the annual premium costing 12% of his annual income, the family would have to pay an annual deductible of approximately

$3,000 before the insurance coverage takes effect. After paying the deductible, the family would then have additional out-of-pocket costs for their share of health care costs, typically about 20%. Thus, combining the annual premium, the deductible, and an estimated $1,000 of out-of-pocket costs, the A family would have an annual health care cost of approximately $10,000, or 20% of household income. This coverage clearly is not readily affordable for this family, however one defines affordability.

What if the A family were instead able to obtain health insurance through the exchanges established by the ACA? A household income of $50,000 constitutes 194% of the 2019 FPL for a family of four (Healthcare.gov n.d.). Based on the Health Insurance Marketplace Calculator provided by the Kaiser Family Foundation (n.d.), if the A family did not have access to affordable employer-sponsored coverage, they would be eligible for coverage through the exchanges. The total annual premium for family coverage under a silver-level plan would be $20,481, with PTCs covering $17,376 per year, and the family paying $3,105 per year (about $259 per month). The family's share of the premium would constitute 6.2% of their annual household income. In addition to the annual premium, the family would be responsible for an annual deductible and certain copayments for care utilized.

It should be clear that the A family would be substantially better off purchasing their health insurance through an ACA exchange. However, under current regulations, even though coverage provided by the employer for the family is not affordable under ACA guidelines, coverage for Mr. A alone is "affordable," which makes the family ineligible for PTC and other assistance through the exchanges. This outcome was the result of a simple oversight during the original drafting process of the ACA legislation. It was just an unintended glitch in ACA coverage.

As described by Norris (2019), "Somewhere between two million and 6 million people are impacted by the family glitch. They are disproportionately lower-income, because lower-wage workers have to spend a larger percentage of their income to pay for health insurance if subsidies aren't available." (Norris also points out, "Fortunately for many of the families caught by the glitch, the Children's Health Insurance Program (CHIP) provides coverage for children with household incomes well over 200 percent of poverty in most states.")

The lower-income families impacted by the glitch are as likely to be Democrats as Republicans. A simple amendment to the ACA that redefines "affordable coverage" based on the costs of family coverage for those employees with families needing health insurance is something that should be able to garner backing from congressional Republicans as well as Democrats. Fixing the glitch could be the first rope added to the new bridge across the health care divide.

Addressing Health Care Costs for Older Workers

The 2019 study by Blendon, Benson, and McMurtry reported that approximately 9 in 10 Americans (88%) agreed that "lowering the overall cost of health care" was extremely important. This concern was shared by Republicans and Democrats alike.

One of the groups most affected by these high costs are individuals over the age of 50 but younger than 65 (thus not yet eligible for coverage under Medicare). For example, consider Mr. B, a nonsmoking man age 55. Mr. B is self-employed and makes $50,000 per year—slightly more than 400% of FPL. If he were to acquire health insurance through an ACA exchange, Mr. B would be ineligible for PTC aid, as his income is over the FPL limit. For Mr. B to acquire silver-level coverage in the exchange, he would need to pay $804 per month, or $9,650 per year in premiums. This would constitute 19.3% of his annual before-tax income. If Mr. B were 60 years old, his monthly premium would be $979 per month, constituting 23.5% of his annual income.

Mr. B could also encounter deductibles and copayments up to an additional $8,150 per year, or an additional 16.3% of his income. If he were to require hospitalization or an expensive procedure, he would be hard pressed to pay this amount. He could elect a bronze-level plan with a lower monthly premium ($578 per month at age 55), but this would bring even higher out-of-pocket expenses.

Might Democratic and Republican lawmakers concur that Mr. B should have the option of enrolling in Medicare at age 55, rather than paying a substantial share of his annual income for coverage? Recall from chapter 3 that, in the summer of 2008, Democrat Max Baucus, a member of the Senate Finance Committee, conducted a series of bipartisan discussions in an effort to identify core elements that the new health care legislation needed to address. As part of what he proposed based on these discussions, "the Baucus plan would make health care coverage immediately available to Americans aged 55 to 64 through a Medicare buy-in" (Baucus 2008).

Indeed, a recent public opinion study found strong concurrence for making Medicare available to those age 55 or over. In 2019, the Center for Deliberative Democracy at Stanford University conducted a national study called America in One Room (n.d.). The study "was a national experiment in deliberation by the public about the major issues facing the country." It brought together a representative sample of 523 registered voters from all around the country. The group came together in Dallas, Texas, for four days of "moderated small group discussions and plenary sessions with competing experts and politicians."

Participants were asked to deliberate on alternative policy proposals in five areas, one of which was health care. One of the policy proposals stated, "People aged fifty-five and older should have the option of purchasing Medicare, instead of a private insurance plan." Participants were asked, "How strongly would you oppose or favor this?" By the end of the meeting, 78.5% of all participants were in favor. Breaking participants down by their political party affiliation, 87.8% of Democrats and 69.6% of Republicans favored this option; 17.6% of Republicans were opposed, while an additional 12.8% were neutral, indicating nationwide bipartisan support among this sample of voters.

Could Republican and Democratic lawmakers come to a consensus on this issue? It would seem likely that they could come to this bipartisan agreement with the support of their base. Giving those over age 55 the option of acquiring Medicare without having to spend an unreasonable percentage of their annual income would seem to be one of the policy "ropes" lawmakers could collaboratively weave as part of the footbridge they are constructing across the chasm of US health care.

Addressing the Price of Prescription Drugs

The study by Blendon, Benson, and McMurtry also found that, while 88% of respondents favored lowering overall health care costs, an even larger percentage, 92%, favored lowering the price of prescription drugs. An earlier study conducted by *Politico* and the Harvard T. H. Chan School of Public Health asked a randomly selected, nationally representative sample of 1,014 adults ages 18 and older to identify their top priorities for the new Congress elected in November 2018 and convening in January 2019 (Blendon et al. 2018). The surveyors provided the study participants with a list of 21 potential policy issues the new Congress might address and asked participants to identify those issues they considered "extremely important." The policy issue most often rated as extremely important was "taking action to lower prescription drug prices," with 90% of Democrats and 82% of Republicans prioritizing this issue.

In 2018, Americans spent $335 billion on prescription drugs (Hartman et al. 2020), an increase of 32% over a period of six years. One of the areas in which the federal government spends the most on prescription drugs is Medicare Part D, which offers seniors private coverage options for prescription drugs. In 2018, Part D plans spent a total of $95.2 billion. Of this amount, the federal government contributed $78 billion (Medicare Trustees 2019).

One of the reasons the Part D plan has such high levels of expenditure is a limitation the law placed on Medicare when it was enacted. Under the law, Medicare is explicitly prohibited from negotiating drug prices with pharmaceutical manufacturers. A potential step lawmakers could take collaboratively is to revisit this issue.

In December 2019, the House of Representatives passed H.R. 3, the Elijah E. Cummings Lower Drug Costs Now Act. (Its title is meant to provide a memorial for longtime Congressman Elijah E. Cummings, who died in October 2019.) According to House Speaker Nancy Pelosi, the law "gives Medicare the power to negotiate directly with the drug companies," "makes the lower drug prices negotiated by Medicare available to Americans with private insurance," and "creates a new, $2,000 out-of-pocket limit on prescription drug costs for Medicare beneficiaries" (n.d.). The bill was passed by a vote of 230-192, largely along partisan lines. House Republicans proposed their own bill as an alternative, H.R. 19, the Lower Costs, More Cures Act (Energy and Commerce Republicans 2019).

While H.R. 3 represents a largely partisan approach to reducing pharmaceutical costs, the Senate has developed a bipartisan approach to this task. "In an era of bitter partisanship, Senator Ron Wyden, D-Oregon, and Senator Chuck Grassley, R-Iowa, have consistently shown a willingness to forge bipartisan partnerships. The most recent example of this is The Prescription Drug Pricing Reduction Act" (Cohen 2019). The proposed Senate bill would have two principal components (Sachs 2019): "First, the package redesigns the Medicare Part D benefit structure to provide financial relief to seniors with high out-of-pocket costs (Section 10121), a feature this package has in common with both H.R. 3 and H.R. 19. Seniors' costs would still be capped at $3,100 . . . Second, the package attempts to control price increases for drugs in both Medicare Part B and Part D by requiring additional rebates back to Medicare if drug companies choose to increase their prices more rapidly than inflation."

The Senate bill would take no action to control drug prices in the private insurance market; it would limit its changes to the Medicare Part D program. Although not technically authorizing negotiating drug prices with manufacturers, it would set limits to price increases based on the rate of inflation. While the Trump administration expressed its strong opposition to H.R. 3, it endorsed the proposed Senate bill.

An analysis by the Kaiser Family Foundation (Cubanski et al. 2020) found that the House and Senate bills have some key elements in common. Both would address the public concern over high drug prices under Medicare Part D. A decision in the House to work with House and Senate Republicans to enact a bill to address Part D prices, while leaving price controls in the private market for another day, would have a strong chance of gaining approval. This would provide the third "rope" with which to weave the initial footbridge across the partisan divide over health care.

Coming to a Consensus on Cost-Sharing Reductions

In chapter 6 I described the efforts by the Republican-led House of Representatives to block federal payment of cost-sharing reduction subsidies. When President Trump took office, the House and the president came to an agreement to end these payments to insurers.

The outcome of the termination of these payments was silver loading, with substantial increases in premiums for silver-level plans sold on the ACA exchanges. An unintended consequence of the cessation of CSR payments was an increase in federal expenditures. A report by the Congressional Budget Office (2017) indicated that the net effect of ending the CSR payments to insurers would be an increase in the federal deficit by $247 billion for the period of 2017–26. While the reduction of CSR payments would total $118 billion, the increase in PTC subsidy for those with incomes less than 400% of FPL would be $365 billion, due to the marked increase in silver-level premiums.

Over 100 insurance companies filed a class-action lawsuit against the federal government for payment of CSR subsidies that had been denied by the Trump administration. "On October 22, 2019, Judge Margaret M. Sweeney issued a final decision in a class action lawsuit brought by insurers over unpaid cost-sharing reduction (CSR) payments. She held that the estimated 100 insurers in the class are owed nearly $1.6 billion in unpaid CSRs for 2017 and 2018" (Keith 2019). The Trump administration appealed the ruling, with the appeals court hearing oral arguments on January 9, 2020. As I described in chapter 6, on August 14, 2020, the court ruled that the federal government has an "unambiguous obligation" to reimburse insurance companies for the CSRs they had made.

While the ruling by the Appeals court mandated that the federal government reimburse insurance companies for the costs incurred by providing CSRs, it did not create a means for funding those payments. That would require Congress to amend the ACA to establish a permanent funding allocation for CSR reimbursement. Qiu (2017) reported that, in an effort to reduce the federal deficit by reinstating CSR payments to insurers, "Senator Lamar Alexander, Republican of Tennessee, and Senator

Patty Murray, Democrat of Washington, announced on Tuesday they had reached a compromise bill to continue the subsidies funding for two years. A draft of the legislation indicates that the plan would appropriate the sums 'necessary for payments for cost-sharing reductions' beginning in December 2017 and lasting through 2019." That legislation never received approval during the Trump administration.

With apparent bipartisan consensus among some senators that reinstating the CSR payments to insurers would actually *save* the federal government substantial costs related to PTCs, and with the appeals court ruling requiring payment for CSR subsidies, there would seem to be the potential for Congress to reverse its earlier policy and to reinstate these payments. Bipartisan collaboration to resolve the CSR dispute could create the fourth rope on the new bipartisan bridge.

Adding Bipartisan Handrails to the Bridge to Enhance Safety

Once the villagers in Peru have weaved together the footbridge across the canyon, they then pull two additional ropes across the divide to act as handrails, giving those who cross the bridge something to hold onto. I would suggest that the Senate and the House each take responsibility for one of these ropes by creating a bipartisan committee of party leaders to meet openly on a regular basis to discuss the health care changes they have made and additional changes they might both be able to support.

Recall from chapter 3 that, in the months leading up to the passage of the ACA, Senator Baucus, Democrat of Montana, and Senator Grassley, Republican of Iowa, collaborated to establish both the Senate Finance Committee Roundtable, which met to discuss the options for health care reform on a bipartisan basis, and the Gang of Six senators, who collaborated on drafting legislation. More recently, Senators Grassley and Wyden have worked in a similar bipartisan manner to draft legislation addressing prescription drug costs. As leaders of their party's membership in the Senate Finance Committee, they could agree to invite other senators to form a new Gang of Six (or eight) that would meet regularly with the stated goal of encouraging bipartisanship in the consideration of health care issues.

If both the House majority and minority leaders were to agree to replicate the Senate's bipartisan efforts, they could create a similar forum that would meet on a regular basis to explore bipartisanship. H.R. 19, the Republicans' alternative to H.R. 3, "consists primarily of provisions that had already been adopted on a bipartisan basis by various committees in both chambers" (Sachs 2019). Sachs points out specifically that H.R. 19 has a number of similarities to the bipartisan bill proposed in the Senate. There are health care issues that House Democrats and Republicans agree on, even though there are a number of other things they disagree on. The focus of the new House bipartisan forum would be to focus its efforts not on things the parties disagree on, but rather on things the parties agree on.

If the Senate and the House were to establish these bipartisan forums to continue public discussion of areas of agreement, it would be important for them to continue regardless of which party controls which houses in Congress. If future elections were to bring a change to congressional majorities, the new majority would need to continue to promote continued bipartisan discussions. Only in this way can the handrails remain in place when members of Congress choose to cross the new rope bridge, giving them a sense of security as they do so.

In 1966, Dr. Philip Bonnet, president of the American Hospital Association, described the passage of Medicare as "a fascinating case study of the operation and effectiveness of representative democratic government. At the end, all the lessons that had been learned during the thirty years . . . were woven by the magical arts of political compromise into an impressive tapestry." In writing this book, I have tried to give voice to my own belief in those magical arts. Collaboration by those on both sides of our health care chasm has the very real potential for constructing a bridge across that divide to provide better health care with reduced costs for nearly all Americans.

Summary and Conclusions

Finding the Path to Bipartisanship

THIS BOOK has spanned 75 years of efforts to enact health care reform in the United States. Starting in 1945, with President Truman's failed effort to enact national health insurance, and continuing to 2020, with the Affordable Care Act awaiting the outcomes of yet another Supreme Court review, we have witnessed a seesawing of alternating partisanship and bipartisanship. As this book is published, we find ourselves at the nadir of bipartisan collaboration in health care reform. About a decade earlier, with the initial efforts to design what ended up as the Affordable Care Act (ACA), our country appeared to be in a period of constructive bipartisan collaboration. For several months leaders of both parties worked together in an effort to forge a mutually acceptable plan for the expansion of access to health insurance. This all changed in the spring of 2009 with the advent of the Tea Party; with its rapid growth in the political influence, a new rigid partisanship regarding health insurance and health care reform brought these bipartisan efforts to a standstill.

As I hope this book has made clear, health care reform in the United States has for decades been a tumultuous process. In the 1950s, with the era of McCarthyism, national health care reform was seen as a communist effort to create a system of socialized medicine. The American Medical Association was stridently opposed to any government interference in the private practice of medicine.

Despite this opposition, one population group—low-income seniors— was having an increasingly difficult time affording the ever-rising costs of medical care. The growing national awareness of the need for affordable health insurance for low-income seniors led to a meeting of the minds. The Republican Eisenhower administration reached out to two senior Democrats in Congress, Senator Robert Kerr of Oklahoma and Representative Wilbur Mills of Arkansas, to find a way to provide federal assistance to states to fund health insurance for low-income seniors. As the program was targeting a fairly narrow segment of the population, the AMA offered its support for the Kerr-Mills Act, passed by Congress in 1960.

Passage of the Kerr-Mills Act set in motion a growing national consensus that seniors more generally needed access to affordable health insurance. Senator John Kennedy made government-financed health insurance for seniors more generally a central goal of his 1960 presidential campaign. Once elected president, he worked to establish such a program. His efforts were blocked by a coalition of southern Democrats and conservative Republicans. Following the assassination of President Kennedy in 1963, it fell to President Lyndon Johnson, himself a southern Democrat and former majority leader in the Senate, to continue this effort.

Johnson proved to be a master craftsman of political compromise. In structuring Medicare with separately designed hospital insurance (Part A) and insurance for physician and other outpatient care (Part B), he was able to bring together an extensive coalition of formerly opposed organizations and individuals to pass Medicare in 1965, providing health insurance for all seniors who qualify for Social Security benefits. By including Medicaid as an extension of Kerr-Mills to provide states the option of also covering poor families, he earned the backing of the AMA.

What enabled the leaders of both parties to work together to pass Medicare and Medicaid? Two factors were essential to the formation of the bipartisan consensus: broad national support for a population subgroup that had a genuine need and political leaders with the interpersonal skills and personal commitment to finding compromise solutions. Lyndon Johnson, Wilbur Mills, and a group of senators demonstrated these capacities in passing Medicare and Medicaid.

These same factors came together in 1997 with passage of the State Children's Health Insurance Program, better known as SCHIP. Congress broadly backed SCHIP only a few years after President Clinton failed to pass his Health Security Act. In 1994, Republicans had gained a House majority and installed Newt Gingrich as the Speaker. Gingrich had campaigned on the "Contract with America," a hard-line conservative agenda that established a stark schism between Republicans and Democrats. He brought this intense partisanship to his leadership in the House and to defeating President Clinton's attempt at health care reform.

Despite the partisanship created by Gingrich and his Republican colleagues, we once again had a vulnerable population group—children in low-income working families—who needed health insurance, with sweeping public support to provide it. We also had trusted leaders from both parties coming together to sponsor the SCHIP legislation. Democratic senator Ted Kennedy of Massachusetts partnered with Republican senator Orrin Hatch of Utah to cosponsor the initial bill. Senator John Chafee, Republican of Rhode Island, and Senator Jay Rockefeller, Democrat of West Virginia, joined as co-sponsors. Simultaneously, Representative John Dingell, Democrat of Michigan, and Representative Margaret Roukema, Republican of New Jersey, cosponsored similar legislation in the House.

With the encouragement of President Clinton, leaders of both parties in the House and the Senate worked collaboratively to quickly pass SCHIP. Access to health insurance for these children has become a core element of our health care system, and the program now known as CHIP continues to provide coverage for nearly 10 million children, in addition to the more than 36 million children who have coverage through Medicaid (Medicaid.gov 2020).

Recall from chapter 2 that the original SCHIP funding was due to run out in 2007, 10 years after enactment. With Democratic majorities in both the House and Senate following the elections of 2006, the two parties worked collaboratively to extend funding for an additional 10 years. This legislation was approved by votes of 265-159 in the House and 67-29 in the Senate. For reasons described in the chapter, President Bush vetoed this compromise legislation. The House fell 13 votes short of the two-thirds majority required to override the veto. As a final compromise, Congress approved and President Bush signed a two-year extension of SCHIP funding.

As described in chapter 3, it took the new Congress elected in 2008 only a few weeks to approve the Children's Health Insurance Program Reauthorization Act of 2009 (CHIPRA) by a vote of 290-135 in the House and 66-32 in the Senate. Assuring access to health insurance for children in low-income working families was yet another example of the intersection of a widely recognized social need and a legislative leadership committed to finding a mutually acceptable, bipartisan solution to address it.

In the weeks and months following the enactment of CHIPRA, President Obama worked with leaders of both parties in Congress to begin designing a new approach to increasing access to affordable health insurance for Americans. Senator Max Baucus, the Democratic chairman of the Senate Finance Committee, had been working with colleagues from both parties to develop a bipartisan plan for health insurance reform.

In January 2009, even before President Obama had been inaugurated, Representative Jim Cooper, a Democrat from Tennessee, and Representative Michael Castle, a Republican from Delaware, released their own health care reform proposal. The effort to gain bipartisan support in the House paralleled the effort in the Senate. Groups of senators and representatives from both parties shared a concern for the rising number of Americans who lacked access to affordable health insurance.

By 2009, 46.3 million people, comprising 15.4% of the US population, were uninsured (Cohen, Martinez, and Ward 2010). A few months before the 2008 election, the British journal *The Lancet* (2008, p. 1971) reported in an editorial that, "for many Americans, especially the large number of uninsured and underinsured, the most pressing domestic concern is health care." It appeared that, once again, the confluence of a generally recognized social need for expanded access to health insurance coupled with congressional leaders representing both parties and committed to working collaboratively was in place to enact major health care reform on the level of Medicare in 1965 and SCHIP in 1997.

Enter the Tea Party and Its Influence on Congress

In the spring of 2009, coincident with the bipartisan efforts in Congress to craft health care reform legislation, a group of politically conservative activists founded the Tea Party. The movement focused its opposition to programs that increased taxes or expanded the power of the federal government. It promoted lower taxes, lower federal spending, more state autonomy on setting policies, and increased reliance on market-based approaches to addressing problems.

Over the summer of 2009, the Tea Party began to focus its efforts on recruiting members of Congress to support its goals. One of its principal goals was to prevent the passage of the health reform legislation President Obama and his Democratic colleagues were developing. The proposals being drafted in Congress, despite being bipartisan, were in many ways contrary to the Tea Party's emphasis on limiting federal government control and reducing government spending. By the end of the summer, there was a growing movement among many Republicans in Congress to oppose the proposed health care reform. As I reference in chapter 3, health policy analyst Billy Wynne reported that, by the fall of 2009, "initial bipartisan negotiations led by Finance Committee Chairman Max Baucus had disintegrated, in part due to Tea Party–driven protests at Republican town-halls over the August recess" (2019).

By the time the proposal initially drafted in the Senate Finance Committee following a series of meetings of the bipartisan Gang of Six senators came to the floor, Republican support had largely evaporated. The question facing Senate majority leader Harry Reid was whether he could muster 60 Democratic votes to overcome a filibuster being mounted by Republican Senators. Senate minority leader Mitch McConnell of Kentucky initiated a series of delaying tactics in an effort to block passage of the bill. In the end, by dropping the public option from the proposed legislation and strengthening the restrictions on federal financing of abortions, Reid was able to secure the 60 Democratic votes he needed.

Democrats in Congress succeeded in passing the Affordable Care Act, including the secondary reconciliation bill enacted by the House after approving without amendment the Senate version of the ACA. By the time the final ACA legislation was passed in March 2010, not a single House Republican voted for it. Whereas less than a year before there had been ongoing bipartisan efforts to craft the reform legislation, by the time President Obama signed the ACA into law, there was a stark divide between congressional Republicans and Democrats. Weissert and Weissert (2019, p. 107) describe the outcomes of the reconciliation process in the Senate: "When the health reform bill passed the Senate in 2010, using the reconciliation process to avoid a GOP filibuster, Republican Senators were so angry that they refused to participate in further legislative business, effectively shutting down the Senate."

That divide was also evident among the various states. On March 23, 2010, the same day President Obama signed the ACA, the attorney general of the state of Florida filed a lawsuit in federal court challenging its constitutionality. Twelve other states' attorneys general, principally from Republican-led states, joined Florida as plaintiffs in the lawsuit. They challenged the constitutionality of key aspects of the ACA such as the individual mandate and the mandatory expansion of Medicaid to all people with incomes below 138% of the federal poverty level. To these states, the ACA was a clear example of federal overreach.

The ideological schism triggered by the passage of the ACA was only to deepen and widen over the years following. For the midterm elections in 2010, Tea Party activists focused their attention on regaining control of Congress. They were successful in regaining control of the House with the election of 242 Republicans. While the Democrats were able to maintain a Senate majority, it was reduced from 59 seats to 53 seats. Eric

Cantor, the new Republican majority leader in the House, on the first day of the session introduced the Repealing the Job-Killing Health Care Law Act. About two weeks later, the full House approved the bill by a partisan vote of 245-189. By the summer of 2012, the House had voted 33 times to repeal the ACA. Of course, none of these bills passed the Democratic-controlled Senate.

President Obama was reelected in 2012, with Republicans maintaining their House majority. In the summer of 2013, the House refused to pass a federal budget unless the bill also repealed all funding for the ACA. The Democratic-controlled Senate refused, resulting in a 16-day federal government shutdown beginning on October 1, the first day of the new fiscal year. The bitterness and resentment among many Republicans nationally grew only more strident. Republicans opposed to the ACA filed the *King v. Burwell* lawsuit challenging the authority of the federal government to fund premium assistance tax credits for those enrolled in the ACA through the federal Healthcare.gov exchange. When the suit reached the Supreme Court in 2015, the court for the second time upheld the ACA.

In 2014, the Republican-controlled House filed its own lawsuit against the ACA, challenging the Obama administration's authority to fund the cost-sharing reductions created by the ACA for individuals and families with income below 250% of the poverty level who obtained coverage through the ACA exchanges. Now it wasn't only individual members of Congress who were intransigently opposed to the ACA. It was the House of Representatives itself that was attempting to sue the president in order to weaken or destroy the ACA.

In the elections of November 2014, the Republicans made substantial gains in Congress, expanding their majority in the House and flipping the Senate with a majority of 54 seats. Congressional Republicans could now take coordinated legislative action to weaken or repeal the ACA. With their continuing resentment of the way the Democrats used the reconciliation process in 2010 to gain final passage of the ACA, Republicans in the House introduced the Restoring Americans' Healthcare Freedom Reconciliation Act of 2015. The bill would eliminate many of the central provisions of the ACA. It took the House only one week to enact this legislation and send it on to the Senate. The Senate amended some provisions of the bill and sent it back to the House, where it achieved final approval on January 7, 2016. As expected, President Obama vetoed the legislation the very next day, further inflaming Republicans opposition. Republican efforts, both in Congress as well as nationally, focused on the only means open to them to repeal the ACA: electing a Republican president in November 2016.

Republican efforts to attain this goal adopted a high level of acrimony during the lead-up to the 2016 elections. In chapter 5, I referenced the results of a national poll by Blendon, Benson, and Casey (2016) showing that, while 80% of Democrats had confidence in the ACA, 88% of Republicans believed it was working poorly and should be either repealed or substantially amended.

President Trump had campaigned aggressively for repeal. On January 20, 2017, the day of his inauguration, President Trump issued his first executive order, announcing that "it is the policy of my Administration to seek the prompt repeal of the Patient Protection and Affordable Care Act" (Trump 2017). The House rapidly began work on developing legislation to repeal the ACA. On May 4, the House passed the American Health Care Act of 2017, which would have repealed most of the central components of the ACA. Lacking the votes to pass the House's version of the repeal legislation, Republican majority leader Mitch McConnell introduced the Health Care Freedom Act as an alternative. While not a complete repeal, the legislation would have repealed certain core provisions and weakened others.

Senator John McCain, under treatment for brain cancer, nonetheless came to the floor of the Senate and cast his historic thumbs-down vote defeating McConnell's bill. The Republican efforts to repeal or substantially weaken the ACA ended in failure. President Trump's resentment over this failure to deliver on the executive order he had issued on his first day in office was readily apparent. With most congressional Republicans behind it, the Trump administration began to take a series of administrative steps to weaken the ACA. Two of the most important were the decisions to permanently defund the cost-sharing reductions mandated by the ACA and to defund the risk corridor payments assured to health insurers who entered the marketplace in its initial years. The loss of funding for the cost-sharing reductions resulted in marked destabilization in the ACA exchanges, with premiums for silver-level plans increasing markedly. The termination of the risk corridor payments caused a number of nonprofit health insurance cooperatives to enter bankruptcy and several private insurers to exit the ACA exchanges. The risk corridor payments were eventually reinstated by the Supreme Court in 2020. Likewise, the cost-sharing reductions were reinstated following the decision on August 14, 2020, by the Court of Appeals for the Federal Circuit, as described in chapter 6.

President Trump continued to take additional steps to weaken the ACA, such as expanding private health insurance plans that did not comply with ACA market requirements. The administration also substantially reduced funding for community navigators whose job it was to assist individuals in enrolling in the ACA marketplaces. It was in Congress, however, that the most influential step was taken. In December 2017, Congress approved and President Trump signed the Tax Cuts and Jobs Act of 2017. Although the principal focus of the legislation was a reduction in taxes for many well-off individuals and corporations, the act also repealed the tax penalty created by the ACA as a means of enforcing the individual mandate.

Recall that, as discussed in chapter 4, in the case of the *National Federation of Independent Business v. Sebelius*, the Supreme Court ruled that the individual mandate to purchase health insurance was not permitted under the Constitution, while the tax penalty for opting not to purchase health insurance was permitted. With the tax penalty revoked, that left only the mandate, without any enforcement mechanism. As I described in chapter 8, the state of Texas sued the federal government, claiming that without the tax penalty the individual mandate to purchase health insurance was unconstitutional, and since that one part of the ACA was unconstitutional, the entire ACA was unconstitutional. The federal district court judge in Texas that heard the case agreed.

The state of California and the other original defendants appealed the judge's decision. The federal appeals court heard arguments in the case in August 2019 and issued its ruling in December 2019. As I describe in chapter 8, the court upheld the district judge's ruling that the individual mandate was unconstitutional. Rather than ruling on the severability of the mandate from the remainder of the ACA, the court remanded the case back to the district court judge, advising him "to employ a finer-toothed comb on remand and conduct a more searching inquiry into which provisions of the ACA Congress intended to be inseverable from the individual mandate."

The Supreme Court agreed to review the appeals court ruling during its 2020 term. The Court heard oral arguments on November 10, a week after the election of Joseph Biden as president. A number of comments from the justices focused on the issue of severability. As described by Jost (2020), "It was here that the Court tipped its hand most clearly. Both Chief Justice Roberts and Justice Kavanaugh suggested that they believed the remainder of the ACA was severable from the mandate." The Court will issue its ruling sometime in the spring or summer of 2021.

The deep public divisions over the ACA in the first years of the Trump administration lessened somewhat following the 2018 congressional elections, in which Democrats regained a majority in the House of Representatives. There was a growing national concern that if the ACA were repealed, insurance companies would once again be free to consider preexisting health conditions in setting premiums. There was also a slow but steady shift among states that had initially opted not to expand their state Medicaid program. In 2020, Oklahoma became the 37th state and Missouri became the 38th state to expand Medicaid following voter approval of a citizen ballot initiative in both states to amend their state constitutions to require it.

Bridging the Partisan Divide over the Affordable Care Act

When the ACA was passed in 2010, the Kaiser Family Foundation (KFF) conducted a national poll of the public support for or opposition to the ACA. "The April 2010 KFF Health Tracking Poll found that 46 percent of the public had a favorable opinion of the law and 40 percent had an unfavorable opinion. In that poll the share of Democrats with a favorable view of the ACA was equal to the share of Republicans with an unfavorable one (78 percent each)" (Brodie et al. 2020, p. 463). By 2020, the KFF polls showed that "the ACA is now more popular than at any other point in its ten-year history" (p. 462). Brodie goes on to describe the changes in public perception that have occurred in the 10 years since the ACA was passed. "Although a larger share of the population has come to report feeling helped by the ACA, the overall partisan divide in opinion of the law as a whole has gotten larger over time, not smaller" (p. 464).

By February 2020, overall national favorability for the ACA had peaked at a 55% (Kaiser Family Foundation 2020). Despite a range of benefits that individual Republicans may receive from the ACA, "conservatives see it as embodying numerous government pathologies, including excessive spending, taxation, redistribution, regulation, and violation of individual liberty" (Oberlander 2018, p. 703). Many Republicans "believ[e] the law to be an unwarranted intrusion of the federal government into the health care system" (McIntyre et al. 2020, p. 730).

These authors have identified core aspects of the ACA that have triggered sustained opposition to the ACA among many Republicans:

- Excessive government spending
- Unwarranted levels of taxation
- Unjustified redistribution of resources to lower-income individuals
- Government regulations that violate individual liberty
- An unwarranted intrusion of the federal government into areas that should be decided by the individual states

The sources of this partisanship go deeper than the ACA itself. In the words of Oberlander (2020, p. 476), "The most powerful explanation for the protracted controversy that has engulfed the ACA has little to do with the law itself. Instead, the divisive politics surrounding the ACA reflect broader trends of growing partisanship and polarization in American politics." Sparer (2020, p. 487) reminds us that "establishing a balance of power between states and the federal government has defined the American Republic since its inception. This conflict has played out in sharp relief with the implementation of the Affordable Care Act."

The politics of American health care have always involved balancing federal and state responsibility and authority. While authority for Medicare is concentrated in the federal government, authority for Medicaid rests with the individual states. When the state of Florida and other mostly Republican states filed the lawsuit that was eventually decided by the Supreme Court, the two central complaints were the unreasonable requirement that states expand Medicaid to all poor people and the unjustified and intrusive mandate that individuals purchase health insurance. Such requirements were seen as violating individual liberty and the rights of states. These are perhaps the central issues contributing to the current partisan divide nationally.

Is there a way to bridge this chasm without undermining these core issues? The message I have tried to offer throughout this book is, yes, there is a way. Earlier in this chapter I described what I perceive to be the two factors that enabled President Johnson and Congress to enact Medicare and Medicaid, despite the several years of partisan divide preceding. To achieve that bipartisan consensus, there had to be significant national support for a population group that had a genuine need for improved access to health care, along with political leaders with the interpersonal skills and personal commitment to finding compromise solutions.

In chapter 9, I outlined four potential actions to improve health care that have been shown to have broad national support:

1) fixing the "family glitch" to make premium tax credits available to working families who do not have affordable health insurance options at work;
2) addressing health care costs for older workers by making those age 55 or older eligible to enroll in Medicare;
3) reining in the price of prescription drugs by limiting drug prices, initially for those enrolled in Medicare Part D and eventually for the health insurance market more generally; and
4) coming to a consensus on funding cost-sharing reductions through the ACA exchanges.

These changes would do little to violate individual liberty or impinge on states' authority. The family glitch is experienced by both Republican and Democratic families. Repairing this inadvertent consequence of the legislative language of the ACA would have a far-reaching benefit. Similarly, both opening Medicare to those age 55 and older and controlling the ever-rising price of prescription drugs have broad bipartisan support nationally.

The withholding of funding for the cost-sharing reductions had its intended outcome of destabilizing the health insurance exchanges. It had an even larger unintended effect of substantially increasing federal expenditures. Reinstating this funding would benefit families of all political perspectives and would likely lead to reduced silver-level premiums on the health insurance exchanges. This is especially true in light of the appellate court decision requiring the federal government to reimburse insurance companies for providing cost-sharing reductions. While the court's ruling requires the federal government to reimburse insurance companies for the cost-sharing reductions, it did not specify how the federal government would fund these reimbursements. It seems only reasonable for Congress to amend the ACA to provide an ongoing allocation to fund these mandated reimbursements.

This then leads to the second factor that could reestablish bipartisan collaboration in addressing health care issues: identifying political leaders with the *interpersonal skills* and *personal commitment* to finding compromise solutions. Here is where the metaphor of the Peruvian rope bridge comes in. If congressional leaders of both parties, with the support of the president, had a clear sense that they were not trying to build another Golden Gate Bridge but rather that they were simply trying to weave together a series of ropes that could be drawn across the health care chasm, the leaders from each side could then meet in the middle.

Following the elections of November 2020, we have the very real possibility that President Biden and the leaders in Congress may demonstrate both their interpersonal skills and the personal commitment to finding compromise solutions. With Democrats maintaining leadership in the House and the Senate evenly divided, President Biden may well be able to bring these leaders together.

Herndon (2020) reported in *The New York Times* on the continuing resistance President Biden faced following his election on the part of many supporters of President Trump: "Towering before him is a wall of Republican resistance, starting with Mr. Trump's refusal to concede . . ." However, Joseph Biden brings with him the experience of six terms as a senator and the personal experience of reaching across the aisle to form compromise with his Republican colleagues. As president, Biden remains committed to and capable of reestablishing a sense of bipartisanship among congressional leaders. The Saturday after the November election, Biden appeared on stage as president-elect, along with vice-president-elect Kamala Harris, to address the nation. In his speech, Biden delivered "a message of unity and trying to soothe the extraordinary divisions that defined the last four years in American politics . . ." (Glueck and Kaplan 2020). In his speech, Biden addressed those who had supported President Trump: "But now, let's give each other a chance. It's time to put away the harsh rhetoric, lower the temperature, see each other again, listen to each other again . . . This is the time to heal in America, to restore the soul of America."

As Herndon (2020) described, the continued partisanship expressed by many Trump supporters is "all a far cry from how Mr. Biden framed this election, from the Democratic primary race through his victory speech last weekend. He cast the moment as a chance for the country to excise the political division Mr. Trump has stoked, promising to repair the ideological, racial, and geographic fissures that have grown into chasms since 2016."

It appears that President Biden is well aware of the chasm that has developed in our country. He appears committed to finding a way to bridge that chasm. An important step in this healing process will be to build a bridge across the chasm in American health care. President Biden has the very real potential to work with congressional leaders to build that bridge. Imagine how the leaders of the House and the Senate might respond upon witnessing the successful enactment of the four policy "ropes" of the bridge I describe. Might they respond the way the Peruvian village leaders respond once the new bridge is completed (Great Big Story 2017)?

We always celebrate our new bridge by singing and dancing. I love the bridge, and right now I'm proud and happy that it's being renewed. This bridge makes us all proud. Long live the bridge. May it last forever.

Long live the bipartisan collaboration that enables us to bridge the health care chasm in order to improve health care access and quality for all Americans. May it last forever.

I would like to acknowledge the tremendous support and encouragement I received from the Fellows and staff at the Center for Advanced Study in the Behavioral Sciences (CASBS) at Stanford University. I was Fellow in residence at CASBS for the 2019–20 academic year. It was my time at CASBS that allowed me to delve into the many complexities of our health care system and complete the manuscript for this book. The many conversations and seminars I participated in with the other Fellows contributed substantially to the insights I have tried to convey in the book. While our fellowship year was cut short by the COVID-19 pandemic, the continued online support I received via our remote Zoom meetings was valuable and deeply appreciated.

Preface

Antos JR, Capretta JC. The ACA: Trillions? Yes. A Revolution? No. *Health Affairs* [blog]. April 10, 2020, available at https://www.healthaffairs.org/do/10.1377/hblog20200406.93812/full/.

Bartsch SM, Ferguson MC, McKinnell JA, et al. The Potential Health Care Costs and Resource Use Associated with COVID-19 in the United States. *Health Affairs.* 2020; 39(6), (2020): 1–7. Published online April 23, 2020, available at https://www.healthaffairs.org/doi/10.1377/hlthaff.2020.00426.

Hooper MW, Nápoles AM, Pérez-Stable EJ. COVID-19 and Racial/Ethnic Disparities. *JAMA.* 2020; 323(24): 2466–67.

King JS. Covid-19 and the Need for Health Care Reform. *New England Journal of Medicine.* 2020; 382: e104. DOI: 10.1056/NEJMp2000821

Rice SE. It's Not Enough to "Get Back to Normal"—We Can Rebuild Better. Here's How. *New York Times.* April 29, 2020, A27.

Williams DR, Cooper LA. COVID-19 and Health Equity—a New Kind of "Herd Immunity." *JAMA.* 2020; 323(24): 2478–80.

Introduction

Abelson R. Employer Health Insurance Is Increasingly Unaffordable, Study Finds. *New York Times.* September 26, 2019, p. B4.

Blendon RJ, Benson JM, McMurtry CL. The Upcoming U.S. Health Care Cost Debate—the Public's Views. *New England Journal of Medicine.* 2019; 380: 2487–92.

Levitt L. Medicare for All or Medicare for More? *Journal of American Medical Association.* 2019; 322(1): 16–17.

Oberlander J. Sitting in Limbo—Obamacare under Divided Government. *New England Journal of Medicine.* 2019; 380: 2485–87.

US Senate. Glossary Term—Reconciliation Process. N.d., available at https://www.senate.gov/reference/glossary_term/reconciliation_process.htm, accessed 12/6/19.

Chapter 1. Bipartisanship in Health Care during the Late Twentieth Century

AMA. AMA House Backs Eldercare Program, Asks Study of Kerr-Mills Expansion. *JAMA.* 1965; 191(8): 32–33.

Ball RM. What Medicare's Architects Had in Mind. *Health Affairs.* 1995; 14(4): 62–72.

Bonnet PD. Hospitals and Medicare. *New England Journal of Medicine.* 1966; 275: 995–1000.

Brunn HW. Will It Be Medicare or Will It Be Eldercare? *Minnesota Medicine.* 1965; 48: 401–5.

Cohen WJ. The First 100 Days of Medicare. *Public Health Reports.* 1966; 81(12): 1051–56.

Cohen WJ. Reflections on the Enactment of Medicare and Medicaid. *Health Care Financing Review*; 1985 (Supplement): 3–11.

Langer E. The Doctors' Debate: What to Do When Medicare Comes Is Main Topic at Stormy AMA Session. *Science.* 1965; 149(3680): 164–67.

Langer E. Medicare: Awaiting the Avalanche. *Science.* 1966; 151(3716): 1366–68.

Marmor TR. *The Politics of Medicare.* Chicago: Aldine, 1973.

Moore JD, Smith DG. Legislating Medicaid: Considering Medicaid and Its Origins. *Health Care Financing Review.* 2005; 27(2): 45–52.

New England Journal of Medicine. Editorial—Medicare and the Physician's Responsibility. 1965; 273: 447–48.

Rosenblatt B. Covered: A Week-by-Week Look at the 1965 Politics That Created Medicare and Medicaid. National Academy of Social Insurance. January 10, 2015, available at https://www.nasi.org/discuss/2015/01/covered-week-week-look -1965-politics-created-medicare-medica. NOTE: This history was published in 2015 on the 50th anniversary of the enactment of Medicare and Medicaid. The history lists the occurrences by the date in 1965 in which they took place. References to this site indicate the day the action took place.

Roth RB. Medicare—Its Problems for Practicing Physicians. *JAMA.* 1966; 197(5): 347–59.

Skidmore MJ. Ronald Reagan and "Operation Coffeecup": A Hidden Episode in American Political History. *Journal of American Culture.* 1989; 12(3): 89–96.

Smith EB. Minorities and Medicare. *Journal of the National Medical Association.* 1966; 58(6): 466–67.

Social Security Administration. Social Security History—the Evolution of Medicare. Chapter 3: The Third Round 1943–1950. N.d., available at https://www.ssa.gov /history/corningchap3.html, accessed 9/20/19.

Stewart WH. Surgeon General's Report—Civil Rights and Medicare. *JAMA.* 1966, 196(11): 175.

Ward DF. Are 200,000 Doctors Wrong? *JAMA.* 1965; 191(8): 661–63.

Wayburn E. Medicare and Medi-Cal to Date. *California Medicine.* 1966; 105(4): 305–7.

Wicker T. Medicare's Progress—Blocked 8 Years, It Moves towards Passage as Public Opinion Changes. *New York Times.* March 25, 1965, p. 49.

Chapter 2. Building on the Bipartisanship That Gained Passage of Medicare and Medicaid

Ball RM. Social Security Amendments of 1972: Summary and Legislative History. *Social Security Bulletin.* 1973; 36(3): 3–25.

Ball RM. National Health Insurance: Comments on Selected Issues. *Science.* 1978; 200(4344): 864–70.

Blendon RJ, Edwards JN. Caring for the Uninsured Choices for Reform. *JAMA.* 1991; 265(19): 2563–65.

Blendon RJ, Edwards JN, Hyams AL. Making the Critical Choices. *JAMA*. 1992; 267(18): 2509–20.

Chief E. Need Determination in AFDC Program. *Social Security Bulletin*. 1979; 42(9): 11–21.

Cohen WJ. Reflections on the Enactment of Medicare and Medicaid. *Health Care Financing Review*; 1985(Supplement): 3–11.

CQ Almanac. Hospital Cost Control. 1977, available at http://library.cqpress.com /cqalmanac/document.php?id=cqal77-1203361#499.

CQ Almanac. Catastrophic Health Insurance Bill Enacted. 1988, available at http://library.cqpress.com/cqalmanac/document.php?id=cqal88-1141782.

CQ Almanac. Big Medicare, Medicaid Changes Enacted in Budget Bills. 1997, available at http://library.cqpress.com/cqalmanac/document.php?id=cqal97 -0000181134.

CQ Almanac. Democrats Unable to Overcome Bush Vetoes of Child Health Bills. 2007, available at http://library.cqpress.com/cqalmanac/document.php?id=cqal07 -1006-44904-2047662&type=toc&num=4.

Economist, Technology Quarterly. Innovation's Golden Goose. 2002; 365(8303): 3.

Eggers PW. Medicare's End Stage Renal Disease Program. *Health Care Financing Review*. 2000; 22(1): 55–60.

Ellis GL. PSRO: Current Status of the Professional Standards Review Organization Program. *American Journal of Occupational Therapy*. 1976; 30(6): 370–5.

Enthoven A, Kronick R. A Consumer-Choice Health Plan for the 1990s. *New England Journal of Medicine*. 1989 (a); 320: 29–37.

Enthoven A, Kronick R. A Consumer-Choice Health Plan for the 1990s. *New England Journal of Medicine*. 1989 (b); 320: 94–101.

Enthoven AC. The History and Principles of Managed Competition. *Health Affairs*. 1993; 12 (Supplement 1): 24–48.

Enthoven AC, Kronick R. Universal Health Insurance through Incentives Reform. *JAMA*. 1991; 265(19): 2532–36.

Himmelstein DU, Woolhandler S. A National Health Program for the United States. *New England Journal of Medicine*. 1989; 320: 102–8.

Hinds MD. The 1991 Election: Wofford Wins Senate Race, Turning Back Thornburgh. *New York Times*. November 6, 1991, p. 1.

Lundberg GD. National Health Care Reform—the Aura of Inevitability Intensifies. *JAMA*. 1992; 267(18): 2521–24.

Lyons RD. Carter Proposes Law for Tough Controls on Hospital Charges. *New York Times*. April 26, 1977, p. A1.

Mann C, Rowland D, Garfield R. Historical Overview of Children's Health Care Coverage. *Future of Children*. 2003; 13(1): 30–53.

Oberg CN, Polich CL. Medicaid: Entering the Third Decade. *Health Affairs*. 1988; 7(4): 83–96.

Oberlander JB, Lyons B. Beyond Incrementalism? SCHIP and the Politics of Health Reform. *Health Affairs*. 2009; 28 (Supplement 1) [web exclusive]: w399–w410. https://www.healthaffairs.org/doi/full/10.1377/hlthaff.28.3.w399.

Oliver TR, Lee PR, Lipton HL. A Political History of Medicare and Prescription Drug Coverage. *Milbank Quarterly*. 2004; 82(2): 283–354.

Oxford English Dictionary. N.d., available at https://oed.com, accessed 10/11/19.

Patent and Trademark Law Amendments Act of 1980, Pub. L. No. 96-517, 94 Stat. 3015, December 12, 1980, available at https://uscode.house.gov/statutes/pl/96 /517.pdf.

Peterson MA. Momentum toward Health Care Reform in the U.S. Senate. *Journal of Health Politics, Policy and Law.* 1992; 17(3): 553–74.

Pressman L, Roessner D, Bond J, et al. *The Economic Contribution of University/ Nonprofit Inventions in the United States: 1996–2013.* Prepared for the Biotechnology Industry Organization, March 17, 2015, available at https://www.bio.org /sites/default/files/files/BIO_2015_Update_of_I-O_Eco_Imp.pdf.

Skocpol T. The Rise and Resounding Demise of the Clinton Plan. *Health Affairs.* 1995; 14(1): 66–85.

Starr P. What Happened to Health Care Reform? *American Prospect.* 1995; (20): 20–31, available at http://www.princeton.edu/~starr/20starr.html.

Starr P, Zelman WA. A Bridge to Compromise: Competition under a Budget. *Health Affairs.* 1993; 12(Supplement 1): 7–23.

Stevens AJ. The Enactment of Bayh-Dole. *Journal of Technology Transfer.* 2004; 29(1): 93–99.

Svahn JA, Ross M. Social Security Amendments of 1983: Legislative History and Summary of Provisions. *Social Security Bulletin.* 1983; 46(7): 3–48.

Todd JS, Seekins SV, Krichbaum JA, et al. Health Access America—Strengthening the US Health Care System. *JAMA.* 1991; 265(19): 2503–6.

US Bureau of Labor Statistics. National Longitudinal Survey of Youth, 1979, available at https://www.nlsinfo.org/content/cohorts/nlsy79/other-documentation /codebook-supplement/nlsy79-appendix-2-total-net-family-3.

US Department of Health and Human Services, Office of Research Integrity. Bayh-Dole Act (Public Law: 96–517). N.d., available at https://ori.hhs.gov/content /Chapter-5-Conflicts-of-Interest-bayh-dole-act-public-law-96-517, accessed 10/4/19.

White ER, Zimmerly JG. Professional Standards Review Organizations (PSROs)— What Do They Mean to the Lawyer? *Forum* (American Bar Association. Section of Insurance, Negligence and Compensation Law). 1974; 10(1): 393–403.

Zelizer JE. How Medicare Was Made. *New Yorker,* News Desk. February 15, 2015, available at https://www.newyorker.com/news/news-desk/medicare-made.

Chapter 3. Health Care Reform under the Obama Administration

America's Affordable Health Choices Act of 2009, H.R. 3200, 111th Cong. (2009–2010), available at https://www.congress.gov/bill/111th-congress/house-bill/3200.

Antos J, Wilensky G, Kuttner H. The Obama Plan: More Regulation, Unsustainable Spending. *Health Affairs.* 2008; 27 (Supplement 1): w462–w471.

Baucus M. *Call to Action—Health Reform 2009.* November 12, 2008, available at https://www.finance.senate.gov/imo/media/doc/finalwhitepaper1.pdf.

Bristol N. Obama Allocates Funds for Health-Care Priorities. *Lancet.* 2009; 373(9667): 881–82.

Cooper J, Castle M. Health Reform: A Bipartisan View. *Health Affairs.* 2009; 28(Supplement 1): w169–w172.

Cornyn J. Obamacare Expands Medicaid Program Wrought with Waste, Fraud & Abuse. March 26, 2010, available at https://www.cornyn.senate.gov/content /cornyn-obamacare-expands-medicaid-program-wrought-waste-fraud-abuse.

CQ *Almanac*. CHIP Gets Long-Sought Expansion. 2009 (a), available at http://library.cqpress.com/cqalmanac/document.php?id=cqal09-1183-59550-2251531&type=toc&num=1.

CQ *Almanac*. Landmark Health Care Overhaul: A Long, Acrimonious Journey. 2009 (b), available at http://library.cqpress.com/cqalmanac/document.php?id=cqal09-1183-59550-2251513&type=toc&num=3.

Health Care and Education Reconciliation Act of 2010. H.R. 4872, 111th Congress (2009–2010), available at https://www.congress.gov/bill/111th-congress/house-bill/4872.

Iglehart JK. Expanding Coverage for Children—the Democrats' Power and SCHIP Reauthorization. *New England Journal of Medicine*. 2009; 360(9): 855–57.

Lancet. Editorial—McCain vs Obama on Health Care. June 14, 2008 (a); 371(9629): 1971.

Lancet. Editorial—Obama and Health: Change Can Happen. November 15, 2008 (b). 372(9651): 1707.

McCain JS. Making Access to Quality and Affordable Health Care a Reality for Every American. *JAMA*. 2008; 300(16): 1925–26.

McCaul M. Statement by Congressman McCaul on the Passage of the Democrats' Healthcare Reform Plan. March 21, 2010, available at https://mccaul.house.gov/media-center/press-releases/statement-by-congressman-mccaul-on-the-passage-of-the-democrats.

Obama B. Affordable Health Care for All Americans—the Obama-Biden Plan. *JAMA*. 2008; 300(16): 1927–28.

Obama B. Why We Need Health Care Reform. *New York Times*. August 15, 2009, p. WK9.

Oberlander J. The Partisan Divide—the McCain and Obama Plans for U.S. Health Care Reform. *New England Journal of Medicine*. 2008; 359(8): 781–84.

Oberlander J. Great Expectations—the Obama Administration and Health Care Reform. *New England Journal of Medicine*. 2009; 360(4): 321–23.

Oberlander JB, Lyons B. Beyond Incrementalism? SCHIP and the Politics of Health Reform. *Health Affairs*. 2009; 28 (Supplement 1) [web exclusive]: w399–w410.

Pear R. Senator Takes Initiative on Health Care. *New York Times*. November 11, 2008, p. A18.

Physicians News Digest. AMA Supports H.R. 3200, "America's Affordable Health Choices Act of 2009." July 17, 2009, available at https://physiciansnews.com/2009/07/17/ama-supports-hr-3200-americas-affordable-health-choices-act-of-2009/.

Senate Finance Committee. *Description of Policy Options—Transforming the Health Care Delivery System: Proposals to Improve Patient Care and Reduce Health Care Costs*. April 29, 2009, available at https://www.finance.senate.gov/imo/media/doc/042809%20Health%20Care%20Description%20of%20Policy%20Option.pdf.

Senate Finance Committee. Health Care Reform from Conception to Final Passage—Timeline of the Finance Committee's Work to Reform America's Health Care System. N.d., available at https://www.finance.senate.gov/imo/media/doc/Health%20Care%20Reform%20Timeline.pdf, accessed 10/18/19.

Tanne JH. Obama Signs Bill to Insure Four Million More Children in US. *BMJ*. 2009 (a); 338: b498.

Tanne JH. Obama Asks AMA to Support His Healthcare Reform Package. *BMJ*. 2009 (b); 338: b2541: 1522.

Tanne JH. Obama Tries to Defuse Anger over Healthcare Reforms. *BMJ*. 2009 (c); 339: b3385: 417.

Weissert WG, Weissert CS. *Governing Health: The Politics of Health*. 5th ed. Baltimore: Johns Hopkins University Press, 2019.

Woodward C. Obama Taps New Allies and Tackles Age-Old Divisions in Nudging Health Care Reform. *CMAJ*. 2010; 182(2): E111–E113.

Wynne B. How the Senate Got to Sixty on Christmas Eve 2009. *Health Affairs* [blog]. December 20, 2019, available at https://www.healthaffairs.org/do/10.1377/hblog 20191220.858191/full/.

Chapter 4. Growing Congressional Opposition to the Affordable Care Act

Bagley N, Jones DK, Jost TS. Predicting the Fallout from King v. Burwell— Exchanges and the ACA. *New England Journal of Medicine*. 2015; 372: 101–4.

Barr DA. *Introduction to U.S. Health Policy: The Organization, Financing, and Delivery of Health Care in America*. 4th ed. Baltimore: Johns Hopkins University Press, 2016.

Brooks T. The Family Glitch. *Health Affairs*. Health Policy Brief. November 10, 2014, available at https://www.healthaffairs.org/do/10.1377/hpb20141110 .62257/full/.

Competitive Enterprise Institute, Business and Government. N.d., described at https://cei.org/issues/business-and-government.

Dolan AM. *House of Representatives v. Burwell and Congressional Standing to Sue*. Congressional Research Service. September 12, 2016, available at https://fas.org /sgp/crs/misc/R44450.pdf.

Eilperin J, Goldstein A. White House Delays Health Insurance Mandate for Medium-Size Employers until 2016. *Washington Post*. February 10, 2014.

Ethridge E. Obama Administration Issues Defense of Employer Mandate Postponement. The Commonwealth Fund. July 15, 2013, available at https://www .commonwealthfund.org/publications/newsletter-article/obama-administration -issues-defense-employer-mandate-postponement.

Federalist Society. Michael A. Carvin—Partner, Jones Day. N.d., available at https://fedsoc.org/contributors/michael-carvin, accessed 10/28/19.

Florida v. U.S. Department of Health and Human Services, 11th Cir., August 12, 2011, described at https://www.bloomberglaw.com/public/desktop/document/Florida_v _US_Dept_of_Health__Human_Servs_648_F3d_1235_11th_Cir_20?1482430940.

Hall MA. King v. Burwell—ACA Armageddon Averted. *New England Journal of Medicine*. 2015; 373: 497–99.

Harris G. Obama Vetoes Bill to Repeal Health Law and End Planned Parenthood Funding. *New York Times*. January 9, 2016, p. A14.

H.R. 676, 113th Congress (2013–2014), available at https://www.congress.gov/bill /113th-congress/house-resolution/676/summary/36.

Jost TS. Subsidies and the Survival of the ACA—Divided Decisions on Premium Tax Credits. *New England Journal of Medicine*. 2014; 371: 890–91.

Kaiser Family Foundation. *A Guide to the Supreme Court's Decision on the ACA's Medicaid Expansion*. August 2012, available at https://www.kff.org/wp-content /uploads/2013/01/8347.pdf.

Kaiser Family Foundation. Status of State Medicaid Expansion Decisions: Interactive Map. August 17, 2020, available at https://www.kff.org/medicaid/issue-brief /status-of-state-medicaid-expansion-decisions-interactive-map/.

King v. Burwell, 576 U.S. (2015) [syllabus], available at https://www.supremecourt .gov/opinions/14pdf/14-114_qol1.pdf.

King v. Sebelius. No. 3:13-CV-630 (E.D. Va. filed Feb. 18, 2014), available at http://theincidentaleconomist.com/wordpress/wp-content/uploads/2014/02/King-v. -Sebelius-2014.pdf.

Kliff S. The Accidental Case against Obamacare—How a Lawyer, a Law Professor, and a Libertarian Found the Affordable Care Act's Secret Weakness. *Vox.* May 26, 2015, available at https://www.vox.com/2015/3/2/8129539/king-burwell-history.

Musumeci MB. *Are Premium Subsidies Available in States with a Federally-Run Marketplace? A Guide to the Supreme Court Argument in King v. Burwell.* Kaiser Family Foundation. February 25, 2015, available at https://www.kff.org/health -reform/issue-brief/are-premium-subsidies-available-in-states-with-a-federally-run -marketplace-a-guide-to-the-supreme-court-argument-in-king-v-burwell/.

National Federation of Independent Business. N.d., described at https://www.nfib .com/, accessed 10/23/19.

Price T. H.R. 3762—Restoring Americans' Healthcare Freedom Reconciliation Act (Veto Override). N.d., available at https://www.gop.gov/bill/h-r-3762-restoring -americans-healthcare-freedom-reconciliation-act-veto-override/, accessed 10/31/19.

Redhead CS, Kinzer J. *Legislative Actions in the 112th, 113th, and 114th Congresses to Repeal, Defund, or Delay the Affordable Care Act.* Congressional Research Service Report R43289. February 7, 2017 (a), available at https://www .everycrsreport.com/reports/R43289.html.

Redhead CS, Kinzer J. *Implementing the Affordable Care Act: Delays, Extensions, and Other Administrative Actions Taken by the Obama Administration.* Congressional Research Service. April 5, 2017 (b), available at https://crsreports.congress .gov/product/pdf/R/R43474.

SCOTUSblog. National Federation of Independent Business v. Sebelius. 2012, available at https://www.scotusblog.com/case-files/cases/national-federation-of -independent-business-v-sebelius/.

The Federalist Society. Michael A. Carvin—Partner, Jones Day. N.d., available at https://fedsoc.org/contributors/michael-carvin, accessed 10/28/19.

United States Senate. Constitution of the United States, available at https://www .senate.gov/civics/constitution_item/constitution.htm#a1_sec9, accessed 10/30/19.

Weisman J, Parker A. Republicans Back Down, Ending Crisis over Shutdown and Debt Limit. *New York Times.* October 16, 2013, p. A1.

Chapter 5. Efforts to Repeal the Affordable Care Act following the Elections of 2016

American Health Care Act of 2017 [bill history], available at https://www.congress .gov/bill/115th-congress/house-bill/1628/all-actions.

Antos JR, Capretta JC. The Senate Health Care Bill. *Health Affairs* [blog]. June 23, 2017 (a), available at https://www.healthaffairs.org/do/10.1377/hblog20170623 .060797/full/.

Antos JR, Capretta JC. The Graham-Cassidy Plan: Sweeping Changes in a Compressed Time Frame. *Health Affairs* [blog]. September 22, 2017 (b), available at https://www.healthaffairs.org/do/10.1377/hblog20170922.062134/full/.

Antos J, Capretta J, Wilensky G. Replacing the Affordable Care Act and Other Suggested Reforms. *JAMA*. 2016; 315(13): 1324–25.

Blendon RJ, Benson JM, Casey LS. Health Care in the 2016 Election—a View through Voters' Polarized Lenses. *New England Journal of Medicine*. 2016; 375: e37.

Blumberg LJ, Buettgens M, Holahan J. Implications of Partial Repeal of the ACA through Reconciliation. Urban Institute. December 6, 2016, available at https://www.urban.org/research/publication/implications-partial-repeal-aca-through-reconciliation.

Bryan B. Senate Republicans Signal They Plan to Scrap Bill the House Just Passed and Write Their Own. *Business Insider*. May 4, 2017, available at https://www.businessinsider.com/senate-plan-for-healthcare-bill-ahca-2017-5.

Cong. Rec. American Health Care Act of 2017—Motion to Proceed. July 25, 2017, available at https://www.congress.gov/congressional-record/2017/07/25/senate-section/article/S4168-1.

Congressional Budget Office. *How Repealing Portions of the Affordable Care Act Would Affect Health Insurance Coverage and Premiums*. January 17, 2017 (a), available at https://www.cbo.gov/publication/52371.

Congressional Budget Office. *American Health Care Act* [cost estimate]. March 13, 2017 (b), available at https://www.cbo.gov/publication/52486.

Congressional Budget Office. *H.R. 1628, American Health Care Act of 2017* [cost estimate]. May 24, 2017 (c), available at https://www.cbo.gov/publication/52752.

Congressional Budget Office. *H.R. 1628, Better Care Reconciliation Act of 2017* [cost estimate]. June 26, 2017 (d), available at https://www.cbo.gov/publication/52849.

Congressional Budget Office. *Estimate of Direct Spending and Revenue Effects of H.R. 1628, the Healthcare Freedom Act of 2017, an Amendment in the Nature of a Substitute [S.A. 667]*. July 27, 2017 (e), available at https://www.cbo.gov/system/files/115th-congress-2017-2018/costestimate/s.a.667.pdf.

Cowan R, Oliphant J. In Hero's Return, McCain Blasts Congress, Tells Senators to Stand Up to Trump. Reuters. July 25, 2017, available at https://www.reuters.com/article/us-usa-healthcare-mccain-idUSKBN1AA2MB.

Editorial Board. The Senate Hides Its Trumpcare Bill behind Closed Doors. *New York Times*. June 13, 2017 (a), p. A26.

Editorial Board. The Senate's Unaffordable Care Act. *New York Times*. June 23, 2017 (b), p. A26.

Federal Elections Commission. Federal Elections 2016: Election Results for the U.S. President, the U.S. Senate and the U.S. House of Representatives. November 8, 2016, available at https://www.fec.gov/resources/cms-content/documents/federalelections2016.pdf.

Fox L, Lee MJ, Bash D, et al. Senate Won't Vote on GOP Health Care Bill. CNN. September 26, 2017, available at https://www.cnn.com/2017/09/26/politics/health-care-republican-senate-vote/index.html.

Goodnough A, Pear R, Kaplan T. Health Groups Denounce G.O.P. Bill as Its Backers Scramble. *New York Times*. March 9, 2017, p. A1.

Jost T. Examining the House Republican ACA Repeal and Replace Legislation. *Health Affairs* [blog]. March 7, 2017, available at https://www.healthaffairs.org /do/10.1377/hblog20170307.059064/full/.

Jost TS, Lazarus S. Trump's Executive Order on Health Care—Can It Undermine the ACA if Congress Fails to Act? *New England Journal of Medicine*. 2017; 376(13): 1201–3.

Kaiser Family Foundation. 2017. Compare Proposals to Replace the Affordable Care Act, available at https://www.kff.org/interactive/proposals-to-replace-the -affordable-care-act/.

Kasich J, Hickenlooper J, Sandoval B, Wolf T, Walker B, McAuliffe T, Bel Edwards J, Bullock S. Bipartisan Governors Blueprint to Congress. August 30, 2017, available at https://www.scribd.com/document/357716292/Bipartisan-Governors -Blueprint-to-Congress-Aug-30-2017#from_embed.

Long SK, Bart L, Karpman M, et al. Sustained Gains in Coverage, Access, and Affordability under the ACA: A 2017 Update. *Health Affairs*. 2017; 36(9): 1656–62.

Mann C. What Could Reconciliation Mean for Medicaid: Reviewing HR 3762. Georgetown University Center for Children & Families. December 7, 2016, available at https://ccf.georgetown.edu/2016/12/07/what-could-reconciliation -mean-for-medicaid-reviewing-hr-3762/.

McDonough JE. Prospects for Health Care Reform in the U.S. Senate. *New England Journal of Medicine*. 2017; 376(26): 2501–3.

Obama B. Repealing the ACA without a Replacement—the Risks to American Health Care. *New England Journal of Medicine*. 2017; 376(4): 297–99, published online January 6, 2017.

Oberlander J. The End of Obamacare. *New England Journal of Medicine*. 2017; 376(1): 1–3, published online November 16, 2016.

Oberlander J. Repeal, Replace, Repair, Retreat—Republicans' Health Care Quagmire. *New England Journal of Medicine*. 2017 (a); 377(11): 1001–3.

Oberlander J. The Art of Repeal—Republicans' Health Care Reform Muddle. *New England Journal of Medicine*. 2017 (b); 376(16): 1497–99.

Pear R. 13 Men, and No Women, Are Writing New G.O.P. Health Bill in Senate. *New York Times*. May 9, 2017, p. A1.

Pear R, Kaplan T. House Republicans Unveil Plan to Replace Health Law. *New York Times*. March 7, 2017, p. A1.

Pramuk J. GOP Senators Who Blocked Obamacare Repeal Call for Cooperation with Democrats. CNBC. July 28, 2017, available at https://www.cnbc.com/2017 /07/28/mccain-collins-calls-for-bipartisan-health-care-bill-after-blocking -obamacare-repeal.html.

Ramzy A. McCain's Vote Provides Dramatic Moment in 7-Year Battle over Obamacare. *New York Times*. July 28, 2017.

Trump DJ. Minimizing the Economic Burden of the Patient Protection and Affordable Care Act Pending Repeal [Executive Order 13765]. *Federal Register* 82(14); January 20, 2017, available at https://www.govinfo.gov/content/pkg/FR-2017-01 -24/pdf/2017-01799.pdf.

US Department of Health and Human Services. New Report Details Impact of the Affordable Care Act. December 13, 2016, available at https://wayback.archive-it

.org/3926/20170127135924/https://www.hhs.gov/about/news/2016/12/13/new
-report-details-impact-affordable-care-act.html.

Werner E, Fram A. No Repeal for 'Obamacare' in Humiliating Defeat for Trump.
NBC 5 Chicago, published March 24, 2017, updated on March 24, 2017 at
11:20 p.m., available at https://www.nbcchicago.com/news/politics/House-Health
-Care-Vote-AHCA-Trump-Demand-417007763.html.

Wilensky G. The Future of the ACA and Health Care Policy in the United States.
JAMA. 2017 (a); 317(1): 21–22.

Wilensky GR. When Political Imperatives Collide with Policy Objectives. *Milbank
Quarterly.* March 2017 (b).

Wilensky GR. The First Hundred Days for Health Care. *New England Journal of
Medicine.* 2017 (c); 376(25): 2407–9.

Yaver M. Republicans' Secretive Plan for Health Care. *New York Times.* June 9,
2017.

Chapter 6. Attempts by Congress and the Trump Administration to Disrupt ACA Financing

Aron-Dine A. Data: Silver Loading Is Boosting Insurance Coverage. *Health Affairs*
[blog]. September 17, 2019, available at https://www.healthaffairs.org/do/10
.1377/hblog20190913.296052/full/.

Bagley N. Trouble on the Exchanges—Does the United States Owe Billions to Health
Insurers? *New England Journal of Medicine.* 2016; 375(21): 2017–19.

Branham DK, DeLeire T. Zero-Premium Health Insurance Plans Became More
Prevalent in Federal Marketplaces in 2018. *Health Affairs.* 2019; 38(5): 820–25.

Centers for Medicare & Medicaid Services, Center for Consumer Information and
Insurance Oversight. *Risk Corridors Payment and Charge Amounts for Benefit
Year 2014.* November 19, 2015, available at https://www.cms.gov/CCIIO
/Programs-and-Initiatives/Premium-Stabilization-Programs/Downloads/RC-Issuer
-level-Report.pdf.

Centers for Medicare & Medicaid Services, Center for Consumer Information and
Insurance Oversight. *Risk Corridors Payment and Charge Amounts for the 2015
Benefit Year.* November 18, 2016 (a), available at https://www.cms.gov/CCIIO
/Resources/Regulations-and-Guidance/Downloads/2015-RC-Issuer-level-Report
-11-18-16-FINAL-v2.pdf.

Centers for Medicare & Medicaid Services, Center for Consumer Information and
Insurance Oversight. *Risk Corridors Payments for 2015.* September 9, 2016 (b),
available at https://www.cms.gov/CCIIO/Programs-and-Initiatives/Premium
-Stabilization-Programs/Downloads/Risk-Corridors-for-2015-FINAL.PDF.

Centers for Medicare & Medicaid Services, Center for Consumer Information and
Insurance Oversight. Premium Stabilization Programs. 2019, described at https://
www.cms.gov/CCIIO/Programs-and-Initiatives/Premium-Stabilization-Programs/.

Congressional Budget Office. *The Effects of Terminating Payments for Cost-Sharing
Reductions.* August 2017, available at https://www.cbo.gov/system/files/115th
-congress-2017-2018/reports/53009-costsharingreductions.pdf.

Corlette S, Lucia K, Kona M. States Step Up to Protect Consumers in Wake of Cuts
to ACA Cost-Sharing Reduction Payments. The Commonwealth Fund. To the
Point. October 27, 2017, available at https://www.commonwealthfund.org/blog

/2017/states-step-protect-consumers-wake-cuts-aca-cost-sharing-reduction
-payments.

Cox C, Semanskee A, Claxton G, Levitt L. Explaining Health Care Reform: Risk
Adjustment, Reinsurance, and Risk Corridors. Kaiser Family Foundation.
August 17, 2016, available at https://www.kff.org/health-reform/issue-brief
/explaining-health-care-reform-risk-adjustment-reinsurance-and-risk-corridors/.

Crespin D, DeLeire T. As Insurers Exit Affordable Care Act Marketplaces, So Do
Consumers. *Health Affairs.* 2019; 38(11): 1893–901.

Fehr R, Cox C, Levitt L. Data Note: Changes in Enrollment in the Individual Health
Insurance Market through Early 2019. Kaiser Family Foundation. August 21, 2019,
available at https://www.kff.org/private-insurance/issue-brief/data-note-changes-in
-enrollment-in-the-individual-health-insurance-market-through-early-2019/.

Fehr R, Kamal R, Cox C. How ACA Marketplace Premiums Are Changing by
County in 2020. Kaiser Family Foundation. November 7, 2019, available at
https://www.kff.org/health-costs/issue-brief/how-aca-marketplace-premiums-are
-changing-by-county-in-2020/.

Gabel JR, Whitmore H, Green M, et al. The ACA's Cost-Sharing Reduction Plans: A
Key to Affordable Health Coverage for Millions of U.S. Workers. The Commonwealth Fund. October 13, 2016, available at https://www.commonwealthfund.org
/publications/issue-briefs/2016/oct/acas-cost-sharing-reduction-plans-key
-affordable-health-coverage.

Galewitz P. Supreme Court Seems Sympathetic to Insurers in Obamacare Case.
Kaiser Health News. December 10, 2019, available at https://khn.org/news
/supreme-court-seems-sympathetic-to-insurers-in-obamacare-case/.

Galewitz P. Obamacare Co-ops Down from 23 to Final "3 Little Miracles." *Kaiser
Health News.* September 9, 2020, available at https://khn.org/news/obamacare-co
-ops-down-from-23-to-final-3-little-miracles/.

Hulse C. Judge Rules House Can Sue Obama Administration on Health Care
Spending. *New York Times.* September 10, 2015, p. A18.

Jost T. Court Stays Cost-Sharing Reduction Payment Case, Giving Control to New
Administration and Congress (Updated). *Health Affairs* [blog]. December 5, 2016
(a), available at https://www.healthaffairs.org/do/10.1377/hblog20161205
.057823/full/.

Jost T. HHS Vigorously Defends against Insurer Claims for Risk Corridor Payments.
Health Affairs [blog]. October 4, 2016 (b), available at https://www.healthaffairs
.org/do/10.1377/hblog20161004.056939/full/.

Jost T. The Latest Motion in House v. Price Has a Significant Impact on the Future of
CSR Payments. *Health Affairs* [blog]. August 2, 2017 (a), available at https://
www.healthaffairs.org/do/10.1377/hblog20170802.061363/full/.

Jost T. ACA Round-Up: Court Blocks New Contraceptive Coverage Rules; CSR
Case Settlement; Final Tax Bill Released; Open Enrollment Closes. *Health
Affairs* [blog]. December 16, 2017 (b), available at https://www.healthaffairs
.org/action/showDoPubSecure?doi=10.1377%2Fhblog20171215
.665944&format=full.

Jost T. Judge Certifies Insurer's Risk Corridor Case as a Class Action. *Health Affairs*
[blog]. January 4, 2017 (c), available at https://www.healthaffairs.org/do/10.1377
/hblog20170104.058227/full/.

Jost T. Mandate Repeal Provision Ends Health Care Calm. *Health Affairs*. 2018; 37(1): 13–14.

Jost T. Supreme Court to Hear Case on Affordable Care Act's Risk Corridors. The Commonwealth Fund. October 25, 2019, available at https://www.commonwealthfund.org/blog/2019/supreme-court-hear-case-affordable-care-acts-risk-corridors.

Jost T. Court Says Marketplace Insurers Are Entitled to Payments for Reducing Cost-Sharing, but Must Offset Premium Tax Credit Increases. Commonwealth Fund. August 18, 2020, available at https://www.commonwealthfund.org/blog/2020/court-marketplace-insurers-payments-reducing-cost-sharing.

Kaiser Family Foundation. Estimates: Average ACA Marketplace Premiums for Silver Plans Would Need to Increase by 19% to Compensate for Lack of Funding for Cost-Sharing Subsidies. April 6, 2017, available at https://www.kff.org/health-costs/press-release/estimates-average-aca-marketplace-premiums-for-silver-plans-would-need-to-increase-by-19-to-compensate-for-lack-of-funding-for-cost-sharing-subsidies/.

Kaiser Family Foundation. Explaining Health Care Reform: Questions about Health Insurance Subsidies. November 2018, available at https://www.kff.org/health-reform/issue-brief/explaining-health-care-reform-questions-about-health/.

Kamal R, Cox C, Fehr R, et al. How Repeal of the Individual Mandate and Expansion of Loosely Regulated Plans Are Affecting 2019 Premiums. Kaiser Family Foundation. October 26, 2018, available at https://www.kff.org/health-costs/issue-brief/how-repeal-of-the-individual-mandate-and-expansion-of-loosely-regulated-plans-are-affecting-2019-premiums/.

Kamal R, Cox C, Long M, et al. 2019 Premium Changes on ACA Exchanges. Kaiser Family Foundation. October 11, 2018, available at https://www.kff.org/private-insurance/issue-brief/tracking-2019-premium-changes-on-aca-exchanges/?preview_id=258035.

Keith K. Insurers Not Owed Risk Corridor Payments. *Health Affairs* [blog]. June 15, 2018, available at https://www.healthaffairs.org/do/10.1377/hblog20180615.782638/full/.

Keith K. The 2020 Final Payment Notice, Part 1: Insurer and Exchange Provisions. *Health Affairs* [blog]. April 19, 2019 (a), available at https://www.healthaffairs.org/do/10.1377/hblog20190419.213173/full/.

Keith K. ACA Heads Back to Supreme Court. *Health Affairs*. 2019 (b); 38(8): 1257–58.

Keith K. ACA Litigation Round-Up: Risk Corridors, CSRs, AHPs, Short-Term Plans, and More. *Health Affairs* [blog]. May 23, 2019 (c), available at https://www.healthaffairs.org/do/10.1377/hblog20190523.823958/full/.

Keith K. Latest Ruling over Unpaid CSRs. *Health Affairs* [blog]. October 25, 2019 (d), available at https://www.healthaffairs.org/do/10.1377/hblog20191025.570658/full/.

Keith K. Supreme Court Rules That Insurers Are Entitled to Risk Corridors Payments: What the Court Said and What Happens Next. *Health Affairs* [blog]. April 28, 2020 (a), available at https://www.healthaffairs.org/do/10.1377/hblog20200427.34146/full/.

Keith K. Federal Circuit: Insurers Owed Unpaid Cost-Sharing Reductions, Reduced by Higher Premium Tax Credits from Silver Loading. *Health Affairs* [blog].

August 17, 2020 (b), available at https://www.healthaffairs.org/do/10.1377/hblog20200817.609922/full/.

Levitt L, Cox C, Claxton G. *The Effects of Ending the Affordable Care Act's Cost-Sharing Reduction Payments.* Kaiser Family Foundation. April 25, 2017, available at http://files.kff.org/attachment/Issue-Brief-The-Effects-of-Ending-the-Affordable-Care-Acts-Cost-Sharing-Reduction-Payments.

Liptak A. Supreme Court May Back Insurers in $12 Billion Obamacare Case. *New York Times.* December 11, 2019, p. A20.

Liptak A. Supreme Court Rules for Insurers in $12 Billion Obamacare Case. *New York Times.* April 28, 2020, p. B3.

Pear R. House Challenge to Health Law Could Raise Premiums, Administration Says. *New York Times.* May 17, 2016, p. A16.

Pear R, Kaplan T. Trump Threat to Obamacare Would Send Premiums and Deficit Skyward. *New York Times.* August 16, 2017, p. A1.

Qiu L. Calling Cost-Sharing Reduction Payments "a Bailout" Is Misleading. *New York Times.* October 19, 2017, p. A17.

Rae M, Levitt L, Semanskee A. How Many of the Uninsured Can Purchase a Marketplace Plan for Less Than Their Shared Responsibility Penalty? Kaiser Family Foundation. November 9, 2017, available at https://www.kff.org/health-reform/issue-brief/how-many-of-the-uninsured-can-purchase-a-marketplace-plan-for-less-than-their-shared-responsibility-penalty/.

Rasmussen PW, Rice T, Kominski GF. California's New Gold Rush: Marketplace Enrollees Switch to Gold-Tier Plans in Response to Insurance Premium Changes. *Health Affairs.* 2019; 38(11): 1902–10.

Sanger-Katz M. Trump's Attack on Insurer "Gravy Train" Could Actually Help a Lot of Consumers. *New York Times.* October 19, 2017, p. A17.

Trump DJ. Minimizing the Economic Burden of the Patient Protection and Affordable Care Act Pending Repeal [Executive Order 13765]. *Federal Register* 82(14); January 20, 2017, available at https://www.govinfo.gov/content/pkg/FR-2017-01-24/pdf/2017-01799.pdf.

US Centers for Medicare & Medicaid Services. *Trends in Subsidized and Unsubsidized Enrollment.* August 12, 2019 (a), available at https://www.cms.gov/CCIIO/Resources/Forms-Reports-and-Other-Resources/Downloads/Trends-Subsidized-Unsubsidized-Enrollment-BY17-18.pdf.

US Centers for Medicare & Medicaid Services. *Plan Year 2020 Qualified Health Plan Choice and Premiums in HealthCare.gov States.* October 22, 2019 (b), available at https://www.cms.gov/CCIIO/Resources/Data-Resources/Downloads/2020QHPPremiumsChoiceReport.pdf.

Chapter 7. Continuing Efforts to Weaken the Affordable Care Act

Altman D. ACA Mandate Repeal May Be Less Popular Than GOP Thinks. *Axios.* December 5, 2017, available at https://www.axios.com/aca-mandate-repeal-may-be-less-popular-than-gop-thinks-1513388387-0600308e-680b-45c3-a5ee-628ba6f384d8.html.

Barr, DA. *Introduction to U.S. Health Policy: The Organization, Financing, and Delivery of Health Care in America.* 4th ed. Baltimore: Johns Hopkins University Press, 2016.

Becker T, Ponce NA. *Californians Maintain Health Insurance Coverage Despite National Trends.* UCLA Center for Health Policy Research. October 2019, available at https://healthpolicy.ucla.edu/publications/Documents/PDF/2019 /healthinsurance-policybrief-oct2019.pdf.

Congressional Budget Office. *Repealing the Individual Health Insurance Mandate: An Updated Estimate.* November 2017, available at https://www.cbo.gov/system /files/115th-congress-2017-2018/reports/53300-individualmandate.pdf.

Covered California. Navigator Program. May 2019, available at https://hbex .coveredca.com/navigator-program/.

Dietz M, Lucia L, Chen X, et al. *California's Steps to Expand Health Coverage and Improve Affordability—Who Gains and Who Will Be Uninsured?* UCLA Center for Health Policy Research, UC Berkeley Labor Center. November 2019, available at https://healthpolicy.ucla.edu/publications/Documents/PDF/2019 /CAHealthCoverage-report-nov2019.pdf.

Federal Register. Coverage of Certain Preventive Services under the Affordable Care Act. July 14, 2015, available at https://www.federalregister.gov/documents/2015 /07/14/2015-17076/coverage-of-certain-preventive-services-under-the-affordable -care-act.

Frommer R. Efforts to Repeal the Patient Protection and Affordable Care Act. *Columbia Medical Review.* 2018; December 29; 2(1).

Goe CL. Short-Term Plans: No Provider Networks Lead to Large Bills for Consumers. The Commonwealth Fund. To the Point. April 30, 2019, available at https://www.commonwealthfund.org/blog/2019/short-term-plans-large-bills -consumers.

Healthcare.gov. Navigator. N.d., available at https://www.healthcare.gov/glossary /navigator/, accessed 11/20/19.

H.R.1. An Act to Provide for Reconciliation Pursuant to Titles II and V of the Concurrent Resolution on the Budget for Fiscal Year 2018. 115th Congress (2017–2018) [summary], available at https://www.congress.gov/bill/115th -congress/house-bill/1.

Jost T. ACA Round-Up: Court Blocks New Contraceptive Coverage Rules. *Health Affairs* [blog]. December 16, 2017 (a), available at https://www.healthaffairs.org /action/showDoPubSecure?doi=10.1377%2Fhblog20171215.665944&format =full.

Jost T. Second Judge Blocks Contraceptive Coverage Requirement Exemptions. *Health Affairs* [blog]. December 21, 2017 (b), available at https://www .healthaffairs.org/do/10.1377/hblog20171221.300213/full/.

Jost T. Mandate Repeal Provision Ends Health Care Calm. *Health Affairs.* 2018; 37(1): 13–14.

Jost TS. D.C. Circuit Judges Hear Oral Arguments in Association Health Plans Case. The Commonwealth Fund. November 20, 2019, available at https://www .commonwealthfund.org/blog/2019/dc-circuit-judges-hear-oral-arguments -association-health-plans-case.

Kaiser Family Foundation. Poll: Survey of the Non-group Market Finds Most Say the Individual Mandate Was Not a Major Reason They Got Coverage in 2018, and Most Plan to Continue Buying Insurance Despite Recent Repeal of the Mandate Penalty. April 3, 2018, available at https://www.kff.org/health-reform

/press-release/poll-most-non-group-enrollees-plan-to-buy-insurance-despite-repeal
-of-individual-mandate-penalty/.

Kaiser Family Foundation. Enrollment in Individual Market Dips Slightly in Early
2019 after Repeal of Individual Mandate Penalty. August 21, 2019, available at
https://www.kff.org/private-insurance/press-release/enrollment-in-individual
-market-dips-slightly-in-early-2019-after-repeal-of-individual-mandate-penalty/.

Kamal R, Cox C, Fehr R, et al. How Repeal of the Individual Mandate and Expansion of Loosely Regulated Plans Are Affecting 2019 Premiums. Kaiser Family
Foundation. October 26, 2018, available at https://www.kff.org/health-costs/issue
-brief/how-repeal-of-the-individual-mandate-and-expansion-of-loosely-regulated
-plans-are-affecting-2019-premiums/.

Keith K. A Hot Health Policy Summer. *Health Affairs.* 2018; 37(10): 1544–45.

Keith K. Final Rule on Health Reimbursement Arrangements Could Shake Up
Markets. *Health Affairs* [blog]. June 14, 2019 (a), available at https://www
.healthaffairs.org/do/10.1377/hblog20190614.388950/full/.

Keith K. Ninth Circuit Blocks Trump Contraceptive Rules. *Health Affairs* [blog].
October 24, 2019 (b), available at https://www.healthaffairs.org/do/10.1377
/hblog20191024.101370/full/.

Keith K. Litigation Continues; Payment Rule Arrives. *Health Affairs.* 2019 (c); 38(6):
894–95.

Keith K. Supreme Court: No Clear Consensus on Contraceptive Mandate Rules.
Health Affairs [blog]. May 7, 2020, available at https://www-healthaffairs-org
.laneproxy.stanford.edu/do/10.1377/hblog20200507.225892/full/.

Liptak A. Supreme Court Divided over Obamacare's Contraceptive Mandate. *New
York Times.* May 7, 2020 (a), p. A23.

Liptak A. Supreme Court Lets Employers Opt Out of Birth Control Coverage. *New
York Times.* July 9, 2020 (b), p. A1.

Little Sisters of the Poor. N.d., described at http://littlesistersofthepoor.org/our-life
/mission/, accessed 5/13/20.

Morse S. 11 States Sue to Stop Association Health Plans. *Healthcare Finance News.*
July 27, 2018, available at https://www.healthcarefinancenews.com/news/11-states
-sue-stop-association-health-plans.

Ostrov BF, Ibarra AB. With ACA's Future in Peril, California Reins in Rising Health
Insurance Premiums. *Kaiser Health News.* July 9, 2019, available at https://khn
.org/news/with-acas-future-in-peril-california-reins-in-rising-health-insurance
-premiums/.

Palanker D, Kona M, Curran E. States Step Up to Protect Insurance Markets and
Consumers from Short-Term Health Plans. The Commonwealth Fund. May 2,
2019, available at https://www.commonwealthfund.org/publications/issue-briefs
/2019/may/states-step-up-protect-markets-consumers-short-term-plans/.

Pollitz K, Claxton G. Proposals for Insurance Options That Don't Comply with ACA
Rules: Trade-offs in Cost and Regulation. Kaiser Family Foundation. April 18,
2018, available at https://www.kff.org/health-reform/issue-brief/proposals-for
-insurance-options-that-dont-comply-with-aca-rules-trade-offs-in-cost-and
-regulation/.

Pollitz K, Long M, Semanskee A, Kamal R. Understanding Short-Term Limited
Duration Health Insurance. Kaiser Family Foundation. April 23, 2018, available

at https://www.kff.org/health-reform/issue-brief/understanding-short-term-limited
-duration-health-insurance/.

Pollitz K, Tolbert J, Diaz M. Data Note: Limited Navigator Funding for Federal
Marketplace States. Kaiser Family Foundation. November 13, 2019, available at
https://www.kff.org/private-insurance/issue-brief/data-note-further-reductions-in
-navigator-funding-for-federal-marketplace-states/#.

Seervai S, Gunja MZ, Collins SR. Health Plans That Don't Comply with the ACA
Put Consumers at Risk. The Commonwealth Fund. To the Point. November 14,
2019, available at https://www.commonwealthfund.org/blog/2019/health-plans
-that-dont-comply-with-aca-put-consumers-at-risk.

Trump, DJ. Executive Order 13798—Promoting Free Speech and Religious Liberty.
May 4, 2017 (a), available at https://www.govinfo.gov/content/pkg/DCPD
-201700309/pdf/DCPD-201700309.pdf.

Trump, DJ. Executive Order 13813—Promoting Healthcare Choice and Competition
across the United States. October 12, 2017 (b), available at https://www.govinfo
.gov/content/pkg/DCPD-201700742/pdf/DCPD-201700742.pdf.

US Centers for Medicare & Medicaid Services, Center for Consumer Information
and Insurance Oversight. Health Reimbursement Arrangements. N.d., available at
https://www.cms.gov/CCIIO/Programs-and-Initiatives/Health-Insurance-Market
-Reforms/Health-Reimbursement-Arrangements, accessed 11/19/19.

US Department of Labor. ERISA. N.d., available at https://www.dol.gov/general
/topic/health-plans/erisa, accessed 11/21/19.

Volk J, Lucia K. Federal Rule Creating New Health Coverage Option for Employers
Could Destabilize the Individual Market. The Commonwealth Fund. To the
Point. July 24, 2019, available at https://www.commonwealthfund.org/blog/2019
/federal-rule-destabilize-individual-market.

Chapter 8. Two More Attempts to Defeat Key Elements of the Affordable Care Act

Adler JH, Bagley N, Gluck AR, et al. Brief of Amici Curiae, Texas et al v. United States
of America et al and California et al. June 14, 2018, available at https://affordable
careactlitigation.files.wordpress.com/2018/09/adler-bagley-gluck-somin-walsh.pdf.

Alker J. Florida House Committee Approves Bill to Impose Harsh Medicaid Rules
on Low-Income Parents. Georgetown University Center for Children and
Families. March 25, 2019 (a), available at https://ccf.georgetown.edu/2019/03/25
/florida-house-committee-approves-bill-to-impose-harsh-medicaid-rules-on-low
-income-parents/.

Alker J. Why Is Florida's Medicaid Work Reporting Proposal the Harshest in the
Country for Kids and Families? Georgetown University Center for Children and
Families. May 1, 2019 (b), available at https://ccf.georgetown.edu/2019/05/01
/why-is-floridas-medicaid-work-reporting-proposal-the-harshest-in-the-country
-for-kids-and-families/.

Alker J. South Carolina Becomes First State to Impose Harmful Work Requirements
Primarily on Poor Parents. Center for Children & Families, Georgetown University.
December 12, 2019 (c), available at https://ccf.georgetown.edu/2019/12/12/trump
-administration-doubles-down-on-harmful-work-requirements-approves-south
-carolina-to-become-first-state-to-apply-them-exclusively-to-poor-parents/.

Alker J. Appeals Court Strikes Decisively at the Heart of Administrator Verma's Medicaid Agenda. Center for Children & Families, Georgetown University. February 14, 2020, available at https://ccf.georgetown.edu/2020/02/14/appeals-court-strikes-decisively-at-the-heart-of-administrator-vermas-medicaid-agenda/.

Altman D, Kaiser Family Foundation, Brodie M. Trump Is Reading the GOP Base Wrong on the Affordable Care Act. *Axios.* April 3, 2019, available at https://www.axios.com/trump-reading-base-wrong-aca-b6e2521c-d386-4c94-81e8-b018a6aaf3b1.html.

Barr DA. *Introduction to U.S. Health Policy: The Organization, Financing, and Delivery of Health Care in America.* 4th ed. Baltimore: Johns Hopkins University Press, 2016.

Centers for Medicare & Medicaid Services. Arkansas Works. N.d., available at https://www.medicaid.gov/medicaid/section-1115-demo/demonstration-and-waiver-list/?entry=15033, accessed 11/16/19.

Chokshi D, Katz MH. Medicaid Work Requirements—English Poor Law Revisited. *JAMA Internal Medicine.* 2018; 178(11): 1555–57.

de Vogue A, Luhby T. Federal Judge in Texas Strikes Down Affordable Care Act. *CNN Politics,* December 15, 2018, available at https://www.cnn.com/2018/12/14/politics/texas-aca-lawsuit/index.html.

Galewitz P. Federal Judge Again Blocks Medicaid Work Requirements. *Kaiser Health News.* March 27, 2019 (a), available at https://khn.org/news/federal-judge-again-blocks-medicaid-work-requirements/.

Galewitz P. Verma Attacks Critics of Medicaid Work Requirement, Pushes for Tighter Eligibility. *Kaiser Health News.* November 12, 2019 (b), available at https://khn.org/news/verma-attacks-critics-of-medicaid-work-requirement-pushes-for-tighter-eligibility/.

Georgetown University Center for Children and Families. *The Impact of Alabama's Proposed Medicaid Work Requirement on Low-Income Families with Children.* August 2018, available at https://ccf.georgetown.edu/wp-content/uploads/2018/03/AL-Work-Requirements-update-8-18.pdf.

Gluck AR, Graetz MJ. The Severability Doctrine. *New York Times.* March 23, 2012, p. A29.

Goldman AL, Woolhandler S, Himmelstein D, et al. Analysis of Work Requirement Exemptions and Medicaid Spending. *JAMA Internal Medicine.* 2018; 178(11): 1549–52.

Goodnough A. South Carolina Is the 10th State to Impose Medicaid Work Requirements. *New York Times.* December 13, 2019 (a), p. B3.

Goodnough A. Appeals Court Seems Skeptical about Constitutionality of Obamacare Mandate. *New York Times.* July 10, 2019 (b), p. A18.

Goodnough A. Appeals Court Rejects Trump Medicaid Work Requirements in Arkansas. *New York Times.* February 15, 2020, p. A17.

Herndon AW. Many on Right Reject the Call For 'Healing.' *New York Times.* November 15, 2020, Section A, Page 1.

HHS Press Office. HHS Approves New Healthy Indiana Medicaid Demonstration. February 2, 2018, available at https://www.hhs.gov/about/news/2018/02/02/hhs-approves-new-healthy-indiana-medicaid-demonstration.html.

Huberfeld N. *Texas v. US*: Another State-Led Threat to the ACA. BU School of Public Health. July 22, 2019, available at https://www.bu.edu/sph/2019/07/22/texas-v-us-another-state-led-threat-to-the-aca/.

Jost TS. An Autumn Docket Heavy on Health Policy. *Health Affairs*. 2018; 37(11): 1730–31.

Jost TS. The Supreme Court Is Unlikely to Crash the ACA. The Commonwealth Fund [To the Point]. November 13, 2020, available at https://www.commonwealthfund.org/blog/2020/supreme-court-oral-arguments-aca.

Kaiser Family Foundation. Medicaid Waiver Tracker: Approved and Pending Section 1115 Waivers by State. November 11, 2019, available at https://www.kff.org/medicaid/issue-brief/medicaid-waiver-tracker-approved-and-pending-section-1115-waivers-by-state/.

Kaiser Family Foundation. Status of State Action on the Medicaid Expansion Decision. August 17, 2020, available at https://www.kff.org/medicaid/issue-brief/status-of-state-medicaid-expansion-decisions-interactive-map/.

Keith K. Trump Administration Asks Court to Strike Down Entire ACA. *Health Affairs* [blog]. March 26, 2019 (a), available at https://www.healthaffairs.org/do/10.1377/hblog20190326.572950/full/.

Keith K. Fifth Circuit Hears Oral Arguments in *Texas v. United States*. *Health Affairs* [blog]. July 9, 2019 (b), available at https://www.healthaffairs.org/do/10.1377/hblog20190710.648299/full/.

Keith K. Supreme Court Arguments: Even If Mandate Falls, Rest of Affordable Care Act Looks Likely To Be Upheld. Health Affairs [blog]. November 11, 2020, available at https://www.healthaffairs.org/do/10.1377/hblog20201111.916623/full/.

Liptak A. Supreme Court Will Not Rule on Obamacare Appeal. *New York Times*. January 21, 2020, p. A20.

Liptak A. Key Justices Signal Support for Affordable Care Act. *New York Times*. November 11, 2020, Section A, Page 1.

Liptak A, Goodnough A. Supreme Court to Hear Obamacare Appeal. *New York Times*. March 3, 2020, p. A1.

Madubuonwu J, Chen L, Sommers BD. Work Requirements in Kentucky Medicaid: A Policy in Limbo. The Commonwealth Fund. September 27, 2019, available at https://www.commonwealthfund.org/publications/issue-briefs/2019/sep/work-requirements-kentucky-medicaid-policy-limbo.

Mango P. Letter to Carol H. Steckel, Commissioner, Department for Medicaid Services, Commonwealth of Kentucky. November 20, 2018 (a), available at https://www.medicaid.gov/Medicaid-CHIP-Program-Information/By-Topics/Waivers/1115/downloads/ky/ky-health-ca.pdf.

Mango P. Letter approving Kentucky HEALTH 1115 waiver request. November 20, 2018 (b), available at https://www.medicaid.gov/Medicaid-CHIP-Program-Information/By-Topics/Waivers/1115/downloads/ky/ky-health-ca.pdf.

Musumeci MB. A Guide to the Lawsuit Challenging CMS's Approval of the Kentucky HEALTH Medicaid Waiver. Kaiser Family Foundation. January 29, 2018, available at https://www.kff.org/medicaid/issue-brief/a-guide-to-the-lawsuit-challenging-cmss-approval-of-the-kentucky-health-medicaid-waiver/.

Neale B. Opportunities to Promote Work and Community Engagement among Medicaid Beneficiaries. January 11, 2018, available at https://www.medicaid.gov/federal-policy-guidance/downloads/smd18002.pdf.

Price T, Verma S. Letter to governors, March 2017, available at https://www.hhs.gov/sites/default/files/sec-price-admin-verma-ltr.pdf.

Rosenbaum S. The Trump Administration Re-imagines Section 1115 Medicaid Demonstrations—and Medicaid. *Health Affairs* [blog]. November 9, 2017, available at https://www.healthaffairs.org/do/10.1377/hblog20171109.297738/full/.

Rosenbaum S. Experimenting on the Health of the Poor: Inside *Stewart v. Azar. Health Affairs* [blog]. February 5, 2018, available at https://www.healthaffairs.org/do/10.1377/hblog20180204.524941/full/.

Rosenbaum S. "We Have All Seen This Movie Before": Once Again, a Federal Court Vacates HHS Approval of a Medicaid Work Experiment. *Health Affairs* [blog]. August 2, 2019, available at https://www.healthaffairs.org/do/10.1377/hblog20190801.892432/full/.

Rovner J. Federal Appeals Court Strikes Down Portion of Obamacare. *Kaiser Health News*. December 18, 2019, available at https://khn.org/news/federal-appeals-court-strikes-down-portion-of-obamacare/.

Rudowitz R, Musumeci MB, Hall C. February State Data for Medicaid Work Requirements in Arkansas. Kaiser Family Foundation. March 25, 2019, available at https://www.kff.org/medicaid/issue-brief/state-data-for-medicaid-work-requirements-in-arkansas/.

Sanger-Katz M. Democrats Ask Supreme Court for Quick Decision on Obamacare. *New York Times*. January 5, 2020, p. A20.

Schneider A. Judge Blocks Arkansas and Kentucky Medicaid Work Requirement Waivers: What Does This Decision Mean for Other States? Georgetown University Center for Children and Families. March 28, 2019, available at https://ccf.georgetown.edu/2019/03/28/judge-blocks-arkansas-and-kentucky-medicaid-work-requirement-waivers/.

Silvestri DM, Holland ML, Ross JS. State-Level Population Estimates of Individuals Subject to and Not Meeting Proposed Medicaid Work Requirements. *JAMA Internal Medicine*. 2018; 178(11): 1552–55.

Social Security Administration. Compilation of the Social Security Laws. Demonstration Projects, Section 1115. N.d., available at https://www.ssa.gov/OP_Home/ssact/title11/1115.htm, accessed 11/25/19.

Sommers BD, Goldman AL, Blendon RJ, et al. Medicaid Work Requirements—Results from the First Year in Arkansas. *New England Journal of Medicine*. 2019; 381: 1073–82.

Stewart v. Azar. No. 18-152, D.D.C. June 29, 2018, available at https://ecf.dcd.uscourts.gov/cgi-bin/show_public_doc?2018cv0152-74.

Sullivan K, Luhby T. Judge Says Affordable Care Act Will Remain in Effect during Appeal. *CNN Politics*, December 30, 2018, available at https://www.cnn.com/2018/12/30/politics/judge-affordable-care-act-remain-in-effect-appeal/index.html.

Trump DJ. Minimizing the Economic Burden of the Patient Protection and Affordable Care Act Pending Repeal [Executive Order 13765]. *Federal Register* 82(14);

January 20, 2017, available at https://www.govinfo.gov/content/pkg/FR-2017-01
-24/pdf/2017-01799.pdf.

Trump D. @realDonaldTrump. December 14, 2018, 7:07 p.m., available at https://
twitter.com/realdonaldtrump/status/1073761497866747904?lang=en.

Texas v. United States. No. 19-10011, 5th Cir. filed December 18, 2019, available at
https://www.ca5.uscourts.gov/opinions/pub/19/19-10011-CV0.pdf.

Verma S. Remarks by Administrator Seema Verma at the National Association of
Medicaid Directors (NAMD) 2017 Fall Conference. November 7, 2017, available
at https://www.cms.gov/newsroom/fact-sheets/speech-remarks-administrator
-seema-verma-national-association-medicaid-directors-namd-2017-fall.

Wydra EB, Gorod BJ, Frazelle BR, et al. Texas v. United States. Constitutional
Accountability Center, July 2019, available at https://www.theusconstitution.org
/litigation/texas-v-united-states/.

Chapter 9. Bridging the Health Care Chasm

Atlas Obscura. Q'eswachaka Rope Bridge. N.d., available at https://www
.atlasobscura.com/places/last-handwoven-bridge, accessed 1/8/20.

Baucus M. *Call to Action—Health Reform 2009.* November 12, 2008, available at
https://www.finance.senate.gov/imo/media/doc/finalwhitepaper1.pdf.

Blendon RJ, Benson JM, McMurtry CL. The Upcoming U.S. Health Care Cost
Debate—the Public's Views. *New England Journal of Medicine.* 2019; 380:
2487–92.

Blendon RJ, Menschel RL, Kenen J, et al. *Americans' Priorities for the New Congress
in 2019. Politico and Harvard T.H. Chan School of Public Health.* December
2018, available at https://www.politico.com/f/?id=00000168-1450-da94-ad6d
-1ffa86630001.

Bonnet PD. Hospitals and Medicare. *New England Journal of Medicine.* 1966; 275:
995–1000.

Center for Deliberative Democracy. America in One Room: Executive Summary.
N.d., available at https://cdd.stanford.edu/2019/america-in-one-room-results/,
accessed 1/13/20.

Cohen J. Prescription Drug Pricing Reduction Act May Become Law in 2020. *Forbes.*
December 15, 2019, available at https://www.forbes.com/sites/joshuacohen/2019
/12/15/prescription-drug-pricing-reduction-act-may-become-law-in-2020
/#ef36c8d5537c.

Congressional Budget Office. *The Effects of Terminating Payments for Cost-Sharing
Reductions.* August 2017, available at https://www.cbo.gov/system/files/115th
-congress-2017-2018/reports/53009-costsharingreductions.pdf.

Cubanski J, Freed M, Dolan R, Neuman T. What's the Latest on Prescription Drug
Proposals from the Trump Administration, Congress, and the Biden Campaign?
Kaiser Family Foundation. June 30, 2020, available at https://www.kff.org
/slideshow/whats-the-latest-on-prescription-drug-proposals-from-the-trump
-administration-congress-and-the-biden-campaign/.

Dupré J. *Bridges: A History of the World's Most Spectacular Spans.* New York: Black
Dog and Leventhal, 2017.

Energy and Commerce Committee Republicans. Walden, Brady, Foxx, Collins
Introduce Legislation to Lower Drug Costs [press conference]. December 9, 2019,

available at https://republicans-energycommerce.house.gov/news/press-release
/walden-brady-foxx-collins-introduce-legislation-to-lower-drug-costs/.

Great Big Story. The 124-Foot Bridge Woven by Hand. September 5, 2017, available
at https://www.youtube.com/watch?v=JCxnStgZsTw.

Guzman GG. Household Income: 2018. American Community Survey Briefs, US
Census Bureau. September 2019, available at https://www.census.gov/library
/publications/2019/acs/acsbr18-01.html.

Hartman M, Martin AB, Benson J, et al. National Health Care Spending in 2018:
Growth Driven by Accelerations in Medicare and Private Insurance Spending.
Health Affairs. 2020; 39(1): 8–17.

Healthcare.gov. Federal Poverty Level (FPL). N.d., available at https://www
.healthcare.gov/glossary/federal-poverty-level-fpl/, accessed 1/10/20.

Kaiser Family Foundation. 2019 Employer Health Benefits Survey. September 25,
2019, available at https://www.kff.org/health-costs/report/2019-employer-health
-benefits-survey/.

Kaiser Family Foundation. Health Insurance Marketplace Calculator. N.d., available
at https://www.kff.org/interactive/subsidy-calculator/, accessed 1/10/20.

Keith K. Latest Ruling over Unpaid CSRs. *Health Affairs* [blog]. October 25, 2019,
available at https://www.healthaffairs.org/do/10.1377/hblog20191025.570658/full/.

Medicare Trustees. *2019 Annual Report of the Boards of Trustees of the Federal
Hospital Insurance and Federal Supplementary Medical Insurance Trust Funds.*
April 22, 2019, available at https://www.cms.gov/Research-Statistics-Data-and
-Systems/Statistics-Trends-and-Reports/ReportsTrustFunds/Downloads/TR2019.pdf.

Norris L. How Millions Were Left Behind by ACA's "Family Glitch." December 1,
2019, available at https://www.healthinsurance.org/obamacare/no-family-left
-behind-by-obamacare/.

Oberlander J. Sitting in Limbo—Obamacare under Divided Government. *New
England Journal of Medicine.* 2019; 380: 2485–87.

Pelosi N. H.R. 3—the Lower Drug Costs Now Act. N.d., described at https://www
.speaker.gov/LowerDrugCosts, accessed 1/14/20.

Qiu L. Calling Cost-Sharing Reduction Payments "a Bailout" Is Misleading. *New
York Times.* October 19, 2017, p. A17.

Sachs R. Prescription Drug Legislation in Congress: An Update. *Health Affairs*
[blog]. December 12, 2019, available at https://www.healthaffairs.org/do/10.1377
/hblog20191211.802562/full/.

Summary and Conclusions

Blendon RJ, Benson JM, Casey LS. Health Care in the 2016 Election—a View through
Voters' Polarized Lenses. *New England Journal of Medicine.* 2016; 375: e37.

Brodie, M, Hamel EC, Kirzinger A, Altman DE. The Past, Present, and Possible
Future of Public Opinion on the ACA: A Review of 102 Nationally Representa-
tive Public Opinion Polls about the Affordable Care Act, 2010 through 2019.
Health Affairs. 2020; 39(3): 462–70.

Cohen RA, Martinez ME, Ward BW. *Health Insurance Coverage: Early Release of
Estimates from the National Health Interview Survey, 2009.* Division of Health
Interview Statistics, National Center for Health Statistics. 2010, available at
https://www.cdc.gov/nchs/data/nhis/earlyrelease/insur201006.pdf.

Glueck K, Kaplan T. At a Festive Drive-In, Biden Makes Pledge to Govern for All Americans. *The New York Times*. November 8, 2020, Section A, Page 11.

Great Big Story. The 124-Foot Bridge Woven by Hand. September 5, 2017, available at https://www.youtube.com/watch?v=JCxnStgZsTw.

Herndon AW. Many on Right Reject the Call For 'Healing.' *The New York Times*. November 15, 2020, Section A, Page 1.

Jost TS. The Supreme Court Is Unlikely to Crash the ACA. The Commonwealth Fund [To the Point]. November 13, 2020, available at https://www.commonwealthfund.org/blog/2020/supreme-court-oral-arguments-aca.

Kaiser Family Foundation. KFF Health Tracking Poll: The Public's Views on the ACA. May 27, 2020, available at https://www.kff.org/interactive/kff-health-tracking-poll-the-publics-views-on-the-aca/.

Lancet. 2008. Editorial—McCain vs Obama on Health Care. June 14, 2008; 371(9629): 1971.

McIntyre A, Blendon RJ, Benson JM, et al. The Affordable Care Act's Missing Consensus: Values, Attitudes, and Experiences Associated with Competing Health Reform Preferences. *Journal of Health Politics, Policy and Law*. 2020; 45(5): 729–55.

Medicaid.gov. CHIP—Reports & Evaluations. 2020, available at https://www.medicaid.gov/chip/reports-evaluations/index.html.

Oberlander J. The Republican War on Obamacare—What Has It Achieved? *New England Journal of Medicine*. 2018; 379(8): 703–5.

Oberlander J. The Ten Years' War: Politics, Partisanship, and the ACA. *Health Affairs*. 2020; 39(3): 471–78.

Sparer MS. Federalism and the ACA: Lessons for the 2020 Health Policy Debate. *Health Affairs*. 2020; 39(3): 487–93.

Trump DJ. Minimizing the Economic Burden of the Patient Protection and Affordable Care Act Pending Repeal [Executive Order 13765]. *Federal Register* 82(14); January 20, 2017, available at https://www.govinfo.gov/content/pkg/FR-2017-01-24/pdf/2017-01799.pdf.

Weissert WG, Weissert CS. *Governing Health—the Politics of Health*. 5th ed. Baltimore: Johns Hopkins University Press, 2019.

Wynne B. How The Senate Got to Sixty on Christmas Eve 2009. *Health Affairs* [blog]. December 20, 2019, available at https://www.healthaffairs.org/do/10.1377/hblog20191220.858191/full/.